The 24-Hour Rule

The 24-Hour Rule
Living with Alzheimer's

Cheryl Levin-Folio

Copyright © 2016 Cheryl Levin-Folio
All rights reserved.

ISBN: 153731646X
ISBN 13: 9781537316468

TABLE OF CONTENTS

Acknowledgments · vii
Introduction · xi

Chapter 1	Our Love Story ·	1
Chapter 2	Safe Home ·	13
Chapter 3	Food Matters ·	23
Chapter 4	Be Creative ·	47
Chapter 5	Finding a "Buddy" ·	59
Chapter 6	Exercise for Mind and Body · · · · · · · · · · · · · · · · ·	71
Chapter 7	Get Organized ·	93
Chapter 8	A Dog's Unconditional Love · · · · · · · · · · · · · · · ·	111
Chapter 9	Brain Work ·	123
Chapter 10	Care for the Caregiver ·	133
Chapter 11	Decisions About Driving ·	145
Chapter 12	Looking and Feeling Good · · · · · · · · · · · · · · · · · ·	151
Chapter 13	Be Interactive ·	161
Chapter 14	Championing Your Loved One · · · · · · · · · · · · · · ·	173
Chapter 15	Travel Smart ·	189

Chapter 16	Be Proactive: Legal, Financial, and Long-Term Care Planning · 201
Chapter 17	Living the 24-Hour Rule: Your New Normal · · · · 217
	Resources · 229
	Notes · 231

ACKNOWLEDGMENTS

First, many thanks to my family for their love and support; without them this project could not have been possible. Especially to my sister, Joyce, and brother-in-law, Melvyn, you both are always there for me and support my efforts no matter what. I am forever grateful. Also, to my sister-in-law, Toni Lee, and brother-in-law, Freddy, your love and support are sincerely cherished and I am thankful for our loving relationship. A special thank you to Jared and Sammie for being amazing, loving, and compassionate children. I am so very proud of you both. And, more importantly, thank you for letting Michael be a part of your lives. I also wish to thank my very close and wonderful friend Andrea Saewitz for always being there for me and convincing me to retire so that I could spend more time with Michael. Deep appreciation goes to Anne Garr for being a trusted confidant and loyal friend. I am lucky to have you in our life. Thank you to Julie Fohrman for being a longtime good and caring friend; you have truly been a tremendous resource and guide in my "new normal" lifestyle.

A big thank you to Bryan Fields, Michael's best friend and business partner, for your friendship, love, and support; you are forever in my heart. A special thank you to Ronde and Claudia Barber, good friends who helped make it possible for Michael to participate in the clinical trial at Byrd Institute. To my friends at Mountain Sky, the Murray, Glazier, and Morris families, a huge thank you for your support and friendship. A special thanks to Laura Murray, who was a great resource in creating the opportunity for me to write this book. I will always cherish my memories of drunk Jenga, Moscow Mules, and splash ball. Tremendous gratitude goes to my friend Susie Regal Wagner for her encouragement and help in finding my excellent production team.

Much appreciation to my writing partner, Colleen Kapklein, for helping me put into words what I hope will help others care for their loved ones with Alzheimer's. Hats off and many thanks to Beth Nyland for assembling the text, illustrations, and cover to create the book. I am most grateful to Greg Borowski for the excellent, couldn't-be-more-perfect book cover design. Much appreciation to Leslie Levine for her help in coordinating, editing, and spreading the word. I am most grateful to Kelly McNees for her excellent copyediting. Jonathan Plotkin provided guidance and confidence so that I could write our story and, happily, introduced us to art and music, which have opened the doors for Michael to enjoy life with energy and enthusiasm. I am forever grateful that I can continue to watch the twinkle that remains in his eyes.

I especially want to thank Jill Smith and Amanda Smith, MD, for their friendship, support, and the energy they've given to me and Michael throughout our journey; they and the USF Health Byrd Alzheimer's Institute have touched our lives forever. We will always be grateful for being part of the clinical trial that will, hopefully, make medical history.

I am also grateful to Dr. Jeffrey Foreman, a friend and internist I know, for suggesting that I include Michael's signature somewhere in these pages. A significant part of your life begins when you learn how to sign your name. Imagine a time when you could no longer accomplish this simple task. By including Michael's signature at the end of these acknowledgements, I am 1) underscoring that we should never take our ability to sign our names for granted and 2) acknowledging both Michael's struggle and triumph to recall the skills needed to write his signature.

To my Michael, thank you for the years of love, memories, and happiness we have shared together and continue to share. I hope *The 24-Hour Rule*, your legacy, changes the way people view this illness and enriches their lives, even in the face of such an enormous struggle and challenge. Thank you for giving me strength and patience and for always being by my side, encouraging me to continue in our fight. Your confidence in me has helped fuel this journey, and I will always be grateful. You're the love of my life and my inspiration, strength, and best friend. Together, we will fight this illness and help build awareness so that, with others, we can beat Alzheimer's. I love and cherish you today, tomorrow, and forever.

INTRODUCTION

The 24-Hour Rule is based on a philosophy, my husband Michael's, that has carried us through the journey I'm about to share. You'll read about that in Chapter 1: Our Story. But before you get started, here are some loose guidelines for using the book so that you and your loved one with Alzheimer's can benefit in the best ways possible.

First, as with any prescriptive book, you should feel free to read this in the order that makes the most sense to you. You might start at the beginning or rush right over to the closing chapter, Living the 24-Hour Rule. Or you might skim through the pages and settle on a chapter that resonates *today*.

However you read the book, please accept my humble appreciation. If you're caring for someone with Alzheimer's, sitting down to read may be the last thing you want to do. Still, I hope that within these pages you find helpful and relevant information that you can put to use now, and a sense that you are not alone on what can be a painful, exhausting journey. You may already have seen that this difficult journey also can bring out the best in you and perhaps reveal something about your life that you didn't know before.

I hope the book provides solace as well. Managing Alzheimer's can be an overwhelming and exhausting experience, one that can test your strength and patience. Yet fighting this disease—and doing what you can to postpone its ugly effects—can invigorate and energize even the most tired caretaker. Knowledge is power, and *The 24-Hour Rule* is brimming with information adopted from real, everyday, and proven strategies that will help you not only live through the disease but also triumph in your efforts to maintain the highest quality of life for both you and the person with Alzheimer's.

Every step of the way, I wrote the book with you in mind. I've been a survivor all my life, and while I can't unravel the mysteries of this devastating disease, I can push forward with strategies and tips that I am confident will help you get through these tough days, instill integrity and peace into the journey, and maintain your sanity. Everyone deals with this process differently. I hope you never feel as if you need to follow a straight path or apply advice that just doesn't feel right. Your gut, heart, and mind/voice will be working together to help you through each and every day. In other words, as you embark on this journey—one you didn't choose—don't be hard on yourself; that won't help anyone. Every day is different and unpredictable.

In every chapter, you will most definitely get to know me. I am thoroughly open and honest with my feelings about this disease. I also present a rather straightforward point of view when it comes to the changes that occur during the course of the illness—changes in your loved one, of course, but also in the way people and relationships are altered, in good and not so good ways. My hope is that my truth and my personal experience help you create your own new normal as you move through your days as a caretaker.

You'll learn about my loving relationship with Michael throughout the book, but especially in Chapter 1: Our Love Story. I believe it's important for all of us to recognize and honor what came before the disease. Your fond memories, after all, will always be with you. I encourage you to draw on them for strength throughout your journey. I also identify several ways to help you remove as many obstacles as you can. In Chapter 2: Safe Home, for example, I write about the importance of conducting a home safety assessment and offer proven ways to danger-proof your home. You'll read about how to manage medications (time, dosage, storage) and options for purchasing ID jewelry like bracelets from MedicAlert.

Food plays a huge role in the management of Alzheimer's, which is why I included a comprehensive chapter on what to eat, including a little dark chocolate (yay!). For example, I address the benefits of following a Mediterranean diet as well as the MIND diet developed by nutritionists at Rush University Medical Center in Chicago and covered extensively in *The MIND Diet: A Scientific Approach to Enhancing Brain Function and Helping Prevent Alzheimer's and Dementia* by Maggie Moon, MS, RDN. You also will read about what foods to limit or avoid altogether (no sugar and no fried or fast food whenever possible).

One of my favorite chapters is Chapter 5: Finding a "Buddy," because we have had such a positive experience with Lee, Michael's buddy. A buddy is someone you actually pay to be a companion for your loved one: a friend with no judgments, just a willingness to spend quality time with someone suffering from Alzheimer's. Another key chapter is one that focuses on exercise. You'll learn how to incorporate movement into your daily lives and see how movement can bring out the best in us—physically, psychologically, and spiritually.

One of my chief motivations for writing the book was to provide a blueprint for people caring for those with Alzheimer's and a legacy for Michael, so people with the disease know they don't have to lose their dignity or be forgotten but rather remembered in high regard. Chapter 10: Care for the Caregiver goes deep into caring for yourself, which will contribute to the legacy your loved one leaves. Self-care in our busy 24/7 lives is critical and mandatory. Add an Alzheimer's diagnosis to the equation, and taking care of yourself becomes paramount. You'll learn how to incorporate breaks so that you can avoid burnout, and about support groups that will help you stay afloat. I also emphasize the importance of talking about this disease. Keeping it all inside is definitely not good for your physical or mental well-being.

In Chapter 14: Championing Your Loved One, you'll discover more ways to incorporate the illness into your conversations—what it is and how people can help. You'll become one of the many who are doing their best to fight the stigma attached to Alzheimer's and, hopefully, feel a sense of tremendous value in your efforts to educate others. Be the voice and let everyone know it's okay to talk about the disease. In Chapter 15: Travel Smart, you'll pick up solid tips on ways to make getting from here to there efficient and safe. Examples include pre-travel research so that you know exactly what to expect on a particular tour or in a hotel. You'll also see that travel can still be a part of your lives, whether you're headed across town or five states over.

The book would be insufficient without Chapter 16: Be Proactive: Legal, Financial, and Long-Term Care Planning. Here, with as little stress and angst as possible, you'll discover why getting your paperwork in order at the onset of the disease is preferable to putting it off. Finally, the book closes with a discussion of your "new normal," a phrase I never particularly liked but one that is perfect and now part of our lifestyle. I consistently live by Michael's philosophy. The 24-Hour Rule demonstrates a hopeful and positive attitude, something I hope you will keep in mind as you continue your journey. And at the end of the book, you'll also find a few blank pages for notes. I encourage you to read the book with a pen in hand, if possible, so that if something resonates and sparks an idea, you can quickly jot it down without having to race around for something to write on. Lastly, thank you for letting *The 24-Hour Rule* be a part of your life.

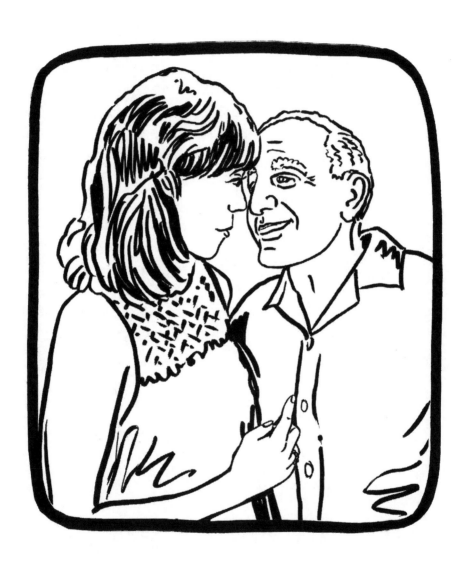

CHAPTER 1

OUR LOVE STORY

This is our story, Michael's and mine. It's about commitment and tenacity and hope. Our story is about patience and respect and support. It's a story of frustration and losses, but also one of strength and resilience.

Our story is about how to live your best life after an Alzheimer's diagnosis. It's a lot of practical information (here's how we did it), and a little bit of inspiration (attitude counts for a lot). This is a story about stepping into a "new normal" nobody wants and making the best of it. This is a story about going through challenges together.

This is a love story.

The 24-Hour Rule

Michael and I had been together a long time but married not even four months when he was officially diagnosed with younger-onset Alzheimer's. When we heard that terrifying diagnosis, here's what we did next: we got on with our lives.

We follow a philosophy Michael used in business for years. I first heard him explain it a long time ago, at a business meeting, and I've never forgotten. Today we use the idea in our day-to-day lives. We've never needed it more than when we first had to face that diagnosis.

The outlook Michael taught me has had a profound impact on our lives, but it can be stated as a simple rule: *when something bad happens to you, you have one day—and one day only—to be sad about it, angry, or whatever.* After that, nothing good will come of wallowing in it; you'll just waste your energy. You have to move forward.

It's tough. You move forward, past it. —Michael

We knew from the start that nothing can cure Alzheimer's. But many things can make living with it better.

From the very beginning of this part of our journey, we were eager to do absolutely everything we could to allow ourselves to live as well as possible for as long as possible. We were proactive people before; we're proactive people now.

The first thing we learned was that the advice from doctors and other professionals, books, and Internet searches could take us only so far. Most information came piecemeal—one tidbit here, another over there. More distressingly, almost everything we found focused on later stages of the disease, described what caregivers (but not patients) could do to help once the situation was dire, and laid out ways to respond to symptoms rather than minimize or delay them. To live fully *now* and preserve as much of our life together as we could, for as long as possible—and to pull everything together in one place so that it might be useful to others—we were going to have to do it ourselves.

And so we did. Over the last few years we've created an extensive, multifaceted program that has kept Michael more engaged and independent, and functioning at a high level for a much longer time than is typically expected in cases like his. The professionals involved with Michael's care have told us many times that they attribute Michael's better-than-expected results to the range of our program and our dedication to sticking with it. Many have told us they wish they could share our program with all their clients or patients, or the caregivers they know. Some have wished they could share it with the classes they teach, preparing the next generation of professional caregivers.

Nothing like this collection of strategies has been available in one resource, until now. Our program has made such a big difference for Michael, and we wanted to make it easy for others on this journey to learn how to live life after an Alzheimer's diagnosis. Our approach also may help anyone with similar challenges to brain performance present in Parkinson's, traumatic brain injury, or other dementias.

Clearly, this journey isn't easy. Nothing about living with Alzheimer's is. But it *is* (relatively) easy to try the things that have worked for us. And the potential upside is huge. There are specific benefits to each of the things we are doing, but I also have discovered that there is value just in having something to *do*.

In a situation that could easily feel hopeless, taking action is one antidote. Education is another—educating yourself and others. Support for the person with Alzheimer's is also a treatment. For us, this means creating an environment that supports Michael's independence for as long as possible. Love, too, is a treatment, and is probably the key ingredient in all that we do.

Our story is all about taking this journey together. More important, I believe it is the secret of our success.

Our story is a love story. But then, isn't all caregiving?

Seashells, Sunsets, and That Damn Scan

Michael and I were married on the beach in Florida, in front of fifty of our closest friends and family. It was perfect. We were at a hotel that held a special place in our hearts, and our ceremony was led by my brother, Barry, and Nina, one of my closet friends. Michael and I exchanged vows we wrote ourselves. Afterward, we walked hand in hand along the beach, as we had for so many years, and collected the most beautiful shells we could find, shells we still display all over our home. The sunset that September day was amazing.

It was the wedding I had dreamed of, and I married the man of my dreams. After a magnificent wedding weekend, and a honeymoon in Key West, we headed back to Chicago, the busy day-to-day with the kids, and the demanding jobs we loved.

We didn't know it then, but everything in our life was about to change.

Over the previous year, Michael had had some heart-related health issues, but a surgical procedure significantly helped, even with the memory issues that this particular kind of heart problem can create. We'd learned that a medication he'd been taking could also interfere with memory, so his doctor changed the prescription. For many months, it appeared that he was getting better.

But at the end of the year, while traveling for business, Michael got lost in the Atlanta airport, a place he'd traveled through many times over the course of his career. To understand what had happened, we decided to see a new doctor, a neurologist. After a whirlwind of appointments and tests, we got the phone call. The amyloid beta PET scan was conclusive: Michael had Alzheimer's.

He was only fifty-six years old.

This was devastating news, of course—a total nightmare. We had a long and emotional discussion lying in bed together. Michael reacted strongly. I felt scared. We were both sad and crying. I'll never forget Michael telling me, "You didn't sign up for this." I told *him* that's not the way it works. We've never run away from anything, I said to him, and we're not starting now. "I love you," I said, "and I would never leave you."

That day, crying together in the dark, we didn't know what lay ahead, but we did agree on one important and fundamental fact: whatever the path, wherever it took us, we would walk it together.

We love each other, and it helps. You have to have that. —Michael

---

What Now?

The day our doctor called with the official diagnosis, I could barely focus. I think I was in shock. But he asked me to schedule an appointment to come in so we could discuss next steps. Once I collected myself, the day of the appointment couldn't come soon enough for me. Michael and I took our 24 hours, for sure, but then we were eager to *do* something. But what?

It was a hard meeting. The doctor told Michael to retire. He also suggested that he stop driving (which he did, six months later). He laid out what changes we could expect over time. He prescribed medications and explained that, although they were the best available, they could only control symptoms, not slow progression of the disease, and definitely couldn't stop, reverse, or cure the disease. Nothing could.

Beyond the medicines, the doctor suggested following a Mediterranean diet and staying active. He recommended keeping the brain active but didn't explain how to do so. Many people recommend doing crossword puzzles, but was that really the best thing to do? It couldn't be the only thing, could it?

I love our neurologist and am grateful for all his care and support. I know we are in the best medical hands with him and with North Shore Health Systems in the Chicago area. But this wasn't really much of a toolkit for preserving a high quality of life for as long as possible. It is surely good advice, and the best place to start, for people newly facing this diagnosis. We realized it was going to be up to us, however, to figure out the details of *how*, exactly, to eat right and stay physically and mentally active. To reach our goal of living longer in the earlier stages of the disease, and remaining in our familiar life, we would need to reach out to other professionals with specific areas of expertise and then figure out a plan for ourselves.

The basic advice I discovered in the world outside the doctor's office was more about preparing for the future and less about what to do *now*. I learned how to manage the downsides, not what to do to make life better. The information I read warned that things were going to keep getting worse, but offered nothing in the way of how to make—or at least try to make—improvements. Articles and books focused on the end of the line, providing little in the form of a road map for the first, and longest, part of the journey. We were left to wonder, how best to live now? What does a healthy lifestyle mean *now*? How can we preserve as much functionality as possible for as long as possible? How can we make the most of the time we have?

A New Normal

Following the 24-Hour Rule doesn't mean the negative feelings go away, that you should suppress the emotion, or that you should pretend a bad situation isn't bad. It just means that you cannot become totally immersed in it. You have to take action, or you will get stuck. You have to be an advocate rather than a victim.

With this disease, if you believe it is a death sentence, then it is. Those who focus that way have already lost the fight, and it is not an uncommon reaction. But that was *not* something we would accept. We are more when-life-gives-you-lemons-you-make-lemonade people.

Michael and I made a different choice. We know we're still alive and in love, and there is a lot of living to do. So for as long as I can be Michael's advocate, we are going to live as well as possible, creating a positive environment for ourselves. We are going to enjoy our lives and each other. We are going to keep being what we were before we got those scan results: as happy as possible and always in love.

Yes, the details of how we go about it look different now. Our life didn't used to involve two big bubbly dogs, for example, or music lessons. And it used to involve routines that we've had to forgo—working every day and traveling extensively. We are living a "new normal."

We can't go back to the old normal, so we don't waste energy trying to. We focus on making the most of this new normal. We bring forward as much of what we've known and loved as we can for as long as it will work. We explore new things and add the best of them to our lives. We are constantly adjusting. We have our challenges, our ups and our downs, and we know, on a daily basis, that there is no cure. But we are doing whatever we can to keep life productive and fulfilling for as long as time permits. We talk openly about the importance of all the time with each other and our friends and family.

And it's working. I'm writing this just about four years after diagnosis, and although the disease has progressed in some ways, Michael is defying the odds. He's active and engaged—playing golf and tennis, biking, going out with friends and family, playing drums, taking art classes, participating in a clinical trial, supporting Alzheimer's awareness, fundraising for research—and generally having a good time despite the many frustrations that come with challenges to brain function.

I'm convinced it's *because* he does so many things that he is doing as well as he is. The various healthcare professionals we work with have encouraged us to stay with the program we've developed. They stress the importance of maintaining stimulation to the brain in every conceivable way. Michael is a shining example of what can happen when you implement a variety of positive approaches to brain health and Alzheimer's care.

He has his moments, as we all do, and he lives with losses, challenges, and frustrations that you wouldn't wish on anyone. But nine times out of ten, if you look over at Michael, he's got a smile on his face. That's still the same Michael I fell in love with.

That's why we keep going, keep moving, keep adjusting. And that's how we keep finding enjoyment and fulfillment in each day. We just keep *living*.

The person that would never stop…yeah, that's Cheryl! —Michael

How to Read This Book

We've answered questions on the fly about the disease as our story has evolved. Now we've put the best of those answers in this book to share what we've learned. For the most part, the book is addressed to caregivers, but those in the earliest stages of a new diagnosis might want to read all or parts of it too. Both of you will play integral roles in making this plan work.

In this book you'll find chapters on all kinds of ways to stimulate, protect, and enhance the brain to keep it in the best shape possible as it fights this disease. There are chapters on:

- healthy living (diet, exercise)
- safety (driving, making your home safe)
- building positive relationships (a buddy, a dog, socializing, communication)
- organizing your life (lost and found, getting organized, travel, personal care)
- fighting for the cause (participating in research, fighting stigma, raising money, getting involved with your local Alzheimer's Association chapter)
- keeping the brain active (creative and intellectual activities, reminiscing)
- legal and financial planning and protection
- caring for the caregiver
- recognizing and understanding what excellent Alzheimer's caregiving looks like

It's not necessary to read the entire book before you start to take action. You can jump right in as soon as something strikes you as helpful or relevant to your particular situation. You can pace yourself and read one chapter at a time, implementing the ideas that appeal to you most. Or, if you're up to it, skip around and try out what best suits you.

The final section includes a list of the best resources we've found for additional assistance and information; you can easily refer to this whenever you are ready to take another step forward.

In the end, though, this is not a one-size-fits-all program. What works for one person might not work the same way for someone else. What works on one day might not work the next. Or what doesn't work one day may be exactly what's needed the next. Treat any plan you make as one in a constant process of revision, and stay flexible. If it ain't broke, don't fix it, of course, but don't be afraid to exclude what's *not* working. Likewise, some months down the line, be open to trying that same tip or strategy again.

We're so glad you've found this book and hope you find our experiences helpful as you walk your path. And we thank you for receiving this book with an open mind, and for being that optimistic person who wants something more than what traditional messages about Alzheimer's suggest you can expect. There's no way out of this situation, but with a little determination you can make the best of your new normal. The recipe requires loads of patience and a positive attitude. Without that, this monumental change in your life may be impossible to manage.

As I look back over our journey, I am stunned, really, by my patience and sense of calm. If you met me five years ago, I don't think you would have seen these traits. It could never have happened without Michael's love and support. He's always brought out the best in me, and he continues to do that today. My love for him helps me be a good caregiver and partner on this road, but his love for me is equally important to the story. Together, we're making our way and finding ways to enjoy each other and our life, even through the tough times. We believe that anyone willing to give the 24-Hour Rule a try can experience the same.

CHAPTER 2

SAFE HOME

For the most part, I generally don't leave Michael home alone. Still, I have put several important measures in place to make sure he is safe. Anything could happen when I am in another room, on the phone, in the bathroom, or anywhere but near Michael. It's impossible for any of us to focus all of our attention on another person 100 percent of the time. And even if you could, you'd still need to implement preventative measures. For example, someone could trip and fall on that loose bathroom area rug, even when you are just a couple of steps away.

This chapter also includes the most important strategies for safety outside the home, and for making sure a person returns home safely if he or she wanders or gets lost.

As I've mentioned, you'll want to create an environment that allows for as much independence as possible while still providing support as needed. The stakes are higher than with, say, household chores or creative activities, so when it comes to safety you have to err on the side of doing too much rather than too little. You need to understand your loved one's limitations and, as geriatric care manager Julie Fohrman says, keep your radar up. Provide support as necessary and empower wherever and whenever you can. Doing so encourages independence and, even more importantly, builds and even sustains self-esteem.

"Proofing" Your Home

You can hire someone to do a home safety assessment for you. In some cases, this might be covered by insurance. If it is feasible for you, it's probably a good investment. An expert is more likely to spot issues you won't necessarily notice, and offer solutions you might not consider. (I didn't think of grab bars in the shower, for example, because I initially thought of that as something for people older than Michael; that was before I learned about the way Alzheimer's can affect balance.) Professionals also might have the necessary products on hand, saving you a lot of shopping trips.

On the other hand, you can take on this task yourself without hiring a pro. Start with clutter: get rid of it. And bring all home maintenance projects up to date. Walk through your home (or the person's home, if you don't share it) and, in each room, pause and ask yourself, *What is the worst-case scenario here?* Look for things that present a risk, keeping in mind that a person with Alzheimer's may have impaired thinking and judgment. Force yourself to think ahead, too, since symptoms can change without notice. Do you need to get a nightlight that goes on automatically once a room is dark, or change to a bulb that's brighter than what you currently have? Do you need a safety gate at the top (and/or bottom) of the stairs? Do you need to keep the knives out of sight instead of visible on the countertop? Do you need "locks" on the stove controls or the faucets? Yes, this process is similar to baby-proofing a home, an endeavor that can feel disheartening. But it will help you in the long run.

Everyone's situation is different. I understand, for instance, that the risk of a stove fire may be more likely in one home versus another. Michael does not initiate cooking, so this is not a worry for us. However, he continues to make his own coffee, but we use a Keurig.

This style of coffeemaker has an automatic shut-off feature and does not pose a safety hazard (though I still check it after breakfast or before we go out). Someone with Alzheimer's who becomes aggressive when stressed might need different precautions than the individual who is more easygoing. It's not always easy to predict what a person with memory issues will do, so you want to imagine what may go awry and then do what you can to avoid that scenario.

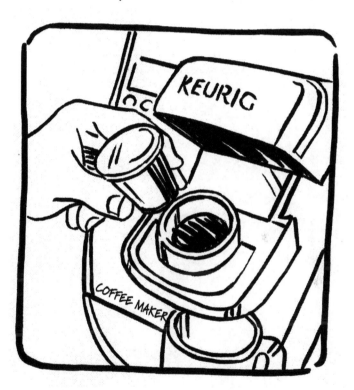

Personal Safety

Creating a safe environment in the home is not only about the physical environment, but also about personal safety. Taking care of general health as best you can is a safety measure. Food can become a source of risk. For example, the chances of choking increase with Alzheimer's. Clothing is another item to consider from a safety perspective. Will slippers increase an individual's chance of falling? Certain styles of shoes should be avoided in general. Grooming products might merit a fresh look too. Does that tube of first-aid cream look too similar to the toothpaste? Would a nail file be a smarter choice than nail scissors? For Michael, we changed right away to an electric razor.

When you create a secure environment, you help make a person with Alzheimer's *feel* safe too.

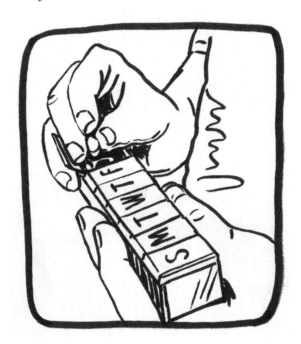

Medication

Michael takes eight pills a day. Getting the right meds in the right dose and at the right time is critical for keeping him healthy and avoiding side effects. Clearly, we don't want to overdose, but we want to avoid undermedicating as well. Plus, keeping track of a complex regimen of medications can be challenging, even before you factor in memory issues, as you may have experienced yourself.

Organization is key. "Strip" boxes for dispensing pills, available at any drugstore, are the first line of defense. I've got one with space for different meds given at different times of day, though our routine is for Michael to take most meds in the morning with his breakfast, a routine that contributes to his safety by ensuring that he gets the right amount of the right stuff.

Michael and I fill the dispenser together; he's there with me when I do it, seeing all the bottles laid out and generally "owning" the process. Michael's at the point where I need to be in charge of getting out the day's dose. I usually just leave it next to his breakfast plate, and he takes over from there: bringing a napkin to the table and laying all the pills out on it. He lays the same pills out in the same pattern every day. Again, the repetition helps him feel in control and makes it less likely we'll forget something.

This is a balance that has shifted, and will continue to shift, over the course of this disease. As much as he can be responsible for, he is. When a task becomes too stressful for Michael, more of the job shifts to me. This is how it goes in our new normal for so many things. With medication, it's a clear matter of safety, so everything needs to be more closely monitored.

I learned the second pillar of our medication safety strategy (and so much more) from Julie Fohrman too: I keep a typed list of current medications at hand for easy reference and take it with me to every doctor's appointment. The list includes the drug's generic name, the dose, the prescribing doctor's name, and what condition the drug is treating. I update this list, without fail, every time there is a change.

The third pillar of medication safety is this: make friends with your pharmacist. From the beginning, I've made a point of speaking personally to Gena at CVS every time I am there, even if just for a minute. I keep her updated, ask her questions (*does this medication make everyone burp so much?*), and solicit her advice. Knowing she is tuned in to the particulars of Michael's situation and that he is more than just an Rx number means she is more likely to catch drug interactions or other problems before they occur. Besides that, she's been extremely helpful in talking to insurance companies more times than I can count. Gena really saved the day the time I accidentally threw out a whole bottle with almost 90 days' worth of medication. That could have been a real nightmare, but she worked with us and our physician to help minimize the mess. Stuff happens, and when it does, I want to be on a first-name basis with the pharmacy staff.

ID Jewelry

Michael wears his "dog tag" and alert bracelet every day. I keep extras on hand for when they get misplaced because I don't want him to go even a day without them. Putting them on is part of our routine, and they help ensure that he can get the specific help he needs, no matter the circumstances. His bracelet is from MedicAlert, and it's paired with the Alzheimer's Association's "Safe Return" program. MedicAlert jewelry identifies key medical conditions, so anyone can tell by looking at Michael's bracelet that he is dealing with "memory impairment"; it also includes emergency contact information and gives emergency personnel access to medical records. Safe Return gives you a 24-hour "emergency response" number to call if a person with Alzheimer's has wandered or gotten lost. Calling that number activates a network of law enforcement agencies and Alzheimer's

Association chapters to facilitate a safe return home. All the relevant professionals—police, firefighters, hospital staff, and so on—will recognize MedicAlert and Safe Return on sight. By the way, MedicAlert offers several stylish-looking variations on their jewelry.

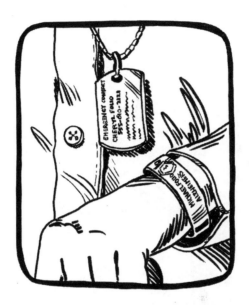

Other companies offer pendants designed for seniors that signal for help in an emergency (like Life Alert), but these are not always effective in cases of memory loss. However, some of the newest versions include GPS technology for use if a person gets lost or wanders.

Be Alarmed

The most important part of being safe at home is simply making sure the person with Alzheimer's *stays* home. Unplanned outings are a safety risk for someone who could become disoriented. And while everyone's situations will vary, the basic strategies are the same:

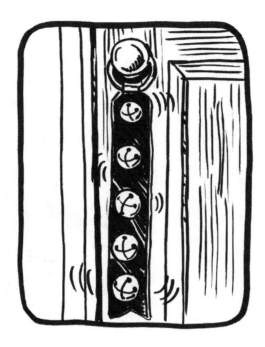

1. Keep all doors locked, even during the day and even when you are at home. Make this a habit.
2. Get a door chime that sounds every time someone opens a door to the outside. Many inexpensive and easy-to-install (no wiring necessary) options are available.
3. An alarm that works similarly to a door chime is a standard part of most home alarm systems. If you have an alarm, leave it on at all times, set to sound when a door opens from inside, but without necessarily alerting the alarm company. Just ask your company how to set it up.

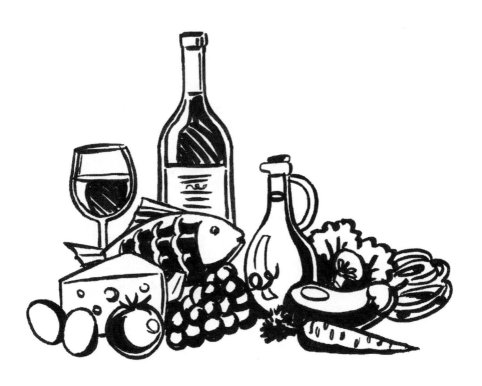

CHAPTER 3

FOOD MATTERS

At our first meeting after the official diagnosis, the doctor gave Michael and me some advice about how to manage Alzheimer's. He talked about medicines, of course, but beyond that he advised Michael to stay active, do puzzles, and follow the Mediterranean diet. He told us that solid research suggests a healthy diet can reduce cognitive decline. For good measure, he recommended taking extra omega-3 in supplement form.

And that was pretty much the sum total of the information he offered about what Michael should be eating. The specifics of how to do this were clearly going to be up to me. I dug in, pulling information from various sources, and eventually figured out a system for getting all the best brain foods into my and Michael's daily diet. The result is this rather long chapter. But don't panic! By the time you finish it, you'll have a clear and easy plan on how to move ahead. And I wholeheartedly agree with the doctor that, along with exercise, eating right is the most important thing we've done to keep Michael living well with Alzheimer's.

After that first doctor's appointment, I went right to the bookstore and bought three cookbooks. The doctor said Mediterranean diet, so I was determined we would follow a Mediterranean diet more carefully than anyone ever had before!

From that day on, we've been all about the fish, olive oil, fruits and vegetables, beans, and nuts, as well as red wine. And even though this isn't often mentioned in Mediterranean diet summaries, we include coffee. Coffee comes with some caveats, which we'll get into later, but still: imagine a lovely café overlooking the sea somewhere in Italy or Greece, where you dine al fresco on equally fresh fish and veggies, and local olives and wine. What could that meal possibly end with but a lovely little cup of antioxidants? Your kitchen, of course, will do just fine as well.

For me, a salad-every-day existence was already familiar territory, but Michael, though always a fan of fish and seafood, was really more of a pasta guy. So it took a little convincing to get him to make the shift. But one of the rules of the Mediterranean diet is—or, at least, should be—to really *enjoy* your food. This is about choosing brain-healthy foods, not depriving yourself in order to stay healthy. So sometimes we treat ourselves to a nice New York Strip or a decadent slice of chocolate cake—just not every day.

Mostly, we just figure out what we could use to replace the foods we had to cross off our list; maybe M&Ms are a no-no, but dark chocolate could scratch that itch just as well. Dress up a turkey burger with all the fixin's, and before long you're not asking "Where's the beef?" On the other hand, sometimes we simply hide the good stuff we don't love in a food that we do. Peanut butter banana smoothie, anyone? You'll never notice the avocado in there, not the way I make it. I swear.

If "the M&M's king," who used to keep bags of the candy squirreled away in his desk drawers, can do it, so can you. This chapter will show you how.

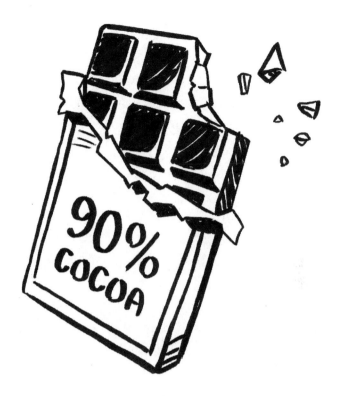

MIND

I went all out with the Mediterranean diet, and I still love those first cookbooks to this day. But I also began searching online for more information on foods that best support brain health. With the Mediterranean diet, we were already focusing on plant-based foods, cutting back on red meat, having fish a few times a week, snacking on nuts, and cooking primarily with extra virgin olive oil.

When I found additional helpful hints, I added in strategies here and there, adapting them to what we like to eat, what we like to cook, and what my kids will eat. Oh, and what might address any other health concerns, such as Michael's high cholesterol levels. It was a continual learning process, and I just kept tinkering. We pretty much cut out sugar. We went mostly gluten free. We switched to eating less dairy and fewer carbohydrates overall than the Mediterranean diet called for per se. I guess you could say we went a little bit Paleo, which essentially includes meat, fish, vegetables, and fruit, and excludes dairy, grain products, and any type of processed food.

But it did become complicated, so I needed to try to simplify. Fortunately, one of my searches led me to the MIND diet, which pulls a lot of this stuff together and groups the ten best foods to include in your diet (and five more you should limit). It even breaks the plan down further to list how many times a day or per week you should eat a given kind of food. This way it's easy to keep track of whether you're getting enough of what's best for your brain.

MIND was developed by nutritionists at Rush University Medical Center in Chicago. In simple terms, it mixes elements of the Mediterranean diet with parts of a diet known as DASH, which was designed to help control high blood pressure. Studies show MIND outperforms either of its two diet inspirations when it comes to protecting brain function. There's good published research demonstrating that eating the MIND way can slow the rate of cognitive decline in people diagnosed with Alzheimer's. A recent study published in the journal *Alzheimer's & Dementia* showed that this diet also has preventative characteristics: people following the MIND diet lowered their risk of Alzheimer's disease by 54 percent, no matter what other risk factors may have been present. It turns out that what's good for the "patient" is good for the caregiver as well.

Dark Chocolate

In my humble opinion, dark chocolate should be its own food group and be added to the MIND diet. Cocoa is full of powerful antioxidants, including catechins, which promote healthy blood flow. It stimulates endorphins, which improve mood. It's a natural stimulant that enhances focus and concentration. The higher the cocoa content, the more benefits (and less sugar) you get, so the darker, the better. We eat it with blueberries, pomegranate, or almonds to double up on brain foods in each delicious bite. I keep 90 percent cocoa bars in the refrigerator at all times because Michael loves chocolate best when it's cold.

The list below shows you what our MIND-inspired, brain-power eating plan looks like. I like the MIND approach: as long as we are getting these ten best foods regularly, and not overindulging in the few *un*helpful foods, I know Michael's brain is getting what it needs most to function as well as it possibly can for him. Beyond that, we just eat a reasonable, healthy diet without sweating too many specifics. There's lots of room for eating all the foods we enjoy, in pretty much infinite variety. (Or *almost* all the foods, anyway. Sorry, cheese.) I'm not counting up calories, hustling to make specific combinations of foods, searching for certain ingredients, or limiting myself to specific recipes. I don't even have to worry about eating something "bad" or "not allowed" because even the limited foods are okay once in a while.

Eating MIND-fully

We make sure to get a serving of these brain-friendly foods at least as often as specified here. (Fish *three* times a week? No problem. Daily blueberries? Help yourself.)

Daily

- Leafy greens, including but not limited to salad greens
- At least one additional vegetable
- Nuts/seeds
- Olive oil
- Whole grains
- Glass of red wine

Every Other Day

- Berries, especially blueberries
- Beans

Weekly

- Fish
- Poultry

Limit or Avoid

The MIND diet isn't an overly strict master. Keep these foods within limits, and you'll still reap all the benefits of the MIND diet:

- Red meat—no more than three servings a week. (Technically, a serving is just four ounces, and most of us habitually down

more than that at a meal and could easily be getting two or three servings in one go.)
- Butter and margarine—no more than one tablespoon a day (including whatever is cooked into your food), and make sure it is grass-fed, which provides more heart-healthy omega-3 fatty acids.
- Cheese—no more than once a week; feta, goat, or mozzarella are the best choices.
- Pastries and sweets—no more than four servings a week.
- Fried or fast food—average less than once a week. Or you can skip these altogether.

How Does This Thing Work?

The Mediterranean and MIND diets have been proven by multiple high-quality studies to help decrease risk of diabetes and many other chronic diseases and even help you avoid some cancers. The diets are especially appealing for protecting heart health—lowering risk of heart disease, high blood pressure, and high cholesterol—and promoting longevity. Some of the most recent studies now show that eating this way also can prevent or delay Alzheimer's and other dementias.

It turns out that what keeps a heart healthy also keeps the brain healthy. Eating Mediterranean/MIND style promotes the good blood circulation that is important to both the heart and the brain. Your brain cells get oxygen and the other fuel they need to function well from your blood. Your blood gets to the brain thanks to the pumping action of your heart. It *doesn't* get there, or not in sufficient quantity anyway, if that pump—and the blood vessels leading to the brain—are damaged. Impaired blood supply to the brain means impaired brain function.

This is NOT the effect we're going for.

Some scientists say the important thing is that the Mediterranean diet is anti-inflammatory, thanks in large part to being naturally rich in omega-3s. Others hail the omega-3s, but for a different reason: the brain needs fats to work, and omega-3s are good fats for the brain. Other camps say what matters most is that the Mediterranean diet keeps cholesterol and blood pressure low and blood vessels healthier. Or maybe it's the large supply of antioxidants this diet delivers. Or the flavonols. Or the vitamins. Or maybe the combination of the three. Or, what's really key could be that obesity increases the risk of Alzheimer's, and the Mediterranean diet helps people get to or keep a healthy weight. And maybe people who are already healthy choose these diets, and volunteer to participate in studies, and that's what makes the difference.

My feeling is this: who cares why it works, exactly, as long as I have my red wine and dark chocolate? It's certainly not going to hurt. The main side effects are increased energy, boosted metabolism, and weight loss. I believe eating well is a big a part of why Michael has maintained his level of functioning for four years and is going strong. And I know I've had more energy, more focus, and more creative thinking myself since we started eating this way.

Ask Your Doctor

Cholesterol contributes to the plaques in the brain associated with Alzheimer's. On the other hand, statin medications used to lower cholesterol levels can cause cognitive impairment. So you need to talk to your cardiologist and/or neurologist about medication for high cholesterol. Michael, for example, changed to a different medication after his Alzheimer's diagnosis.

Good Fats

Your whole body needs good fats. Your heart needs the right fats to stay healthy. But your brain, which is literally *built* out of fats, has a particularly urgent need for fats in order to work at its best. The right fats are also linked to the making of certain neurotransmitters, which are important to learning and memory.

The MIND diet's recommendations emphasize foods rich in healthy fats that nourish the brain: fish, nuts and seeds, and olive oil. That's almost a third of their recommendations overall, which should give you a good idea of how important it is to get the right fats into your body.

So Michael and I snack on nuts almost every day, or put them in a salad, or on oatmeal. We use olive oil almost any time we need oil or fat, including for salad dressings and cooking. We always get our MIND-recommended one serving a week of fish and sometimes more simply because we like it.

We have a few more favorite ways to sneak in even more healthy fats to our diet. We enjoy actual olives—not just their oil—and look to avocado as another excellent source of good fats. Michael doesn't actually *like* avocado, but it is so healthy I disguise it in other foods where it can dispense its brain-healthy fats undetected.

Finally, I recommend coconut, and especially coconut oil, though there's a caveat coming, so keep reading. Coconut provides a somewhat different kind of good fat, because it is saturated fat, which is part of what you're avoiding by limiting red meat and cheese. So why put it on the "good" list? Components of coconut, like caprylic acid and medium-chain triglycerides, are especially good for the brain and brain function. Coconut is *not*, however, good for cholesterol levels in some folks, so you may need to skip it if you are being treated for high cholesterol, like Michael is. And if you are using coconut oil or coconut milk, keep up with your cholesterol checks, just in case.

Healthy fats also can replace *un*helpful fats in your diet. Switch to drizzling a little olive oil over those steamed veggies instead of topping them with a pat of butter (and its saturated fat). This way, you are getting a double bonus: you're eating a healthier food *and* eliminating one that's worse.

Which Fish?

Fish is an excellent source of crucial omega-3 fatty acids, which are anti-inflammatory and otherwise essential for good brain function. The fattier your fish, the more of these omegas you get, so focus on "oily" fish such as:

- *Salmon*
- *Tuna*
- *Anchovies*
- *Mackerel*
- *Sardines*
- *Herring*

We love salmon, especially, but I hold out for buying the wild-caught Pacific kind. Our other favorites—also always wild-caught—include halibut, cod, snapper, and grouper, all of which are in frequent rotation at our house. When you shop, you might want to speak to someone at the fish counter in your grocery store about selections and price specials. Also, remember that canned tuna, herring, and other types of packaged fish are fairly inexpensive and can offer just as much benefit.

Some of these optimal types of fish may be less familiar to you, but a little investigation will turn up appealing ways to incorporate them into your diet. You may just need a reminder about some of these opportunities, like the fact that anchovies are the key to a real Caesar salad—yum! Actually, anchovies are delicious in a lot of dishes, especially when they literally dissolve into the background of a dish like puttanesca sauce. I've always been cautious about having too much sodium in our diet. When I'm cooking, I use sea salt, which is more nutritious than table salt.

Shellfish is usually a good choice as well. Stone crab, when it's in season, is a favorite for both of us. But we have shellfish only rarely as a part of controlling Michael's cholesterol.

Not So Much: Gluten, Sugar, and Dairy

Michael and I have three more things on our list of foods to avoid: gluten, dairy, and sugar. We don't go crazy with it—sometimes we splurge on some whole-wheat pita chips—but, given the choice, we usually opt out.

Some books released in the last couple of years point to gluten, sugar, and dairy as the prime suspects in inflammation, which is the prime suspect in Alzheimer's. Carbs in general are sometimes targeted for this same reason. The studies to back this up 100 percent aren't there yet, but I can say I feel more energetic and less brain-foggy by avoiding these foods, and I think it's part of the dietary change that's been helpful to Michael.

Sugar is as bad for brain health as it is for blood sugar levels. In fact, it's bad for brain health *because* it raises blood sugar levels. In some places, you'll see Alzheimer's referred to as a form of diabetes in the brain. This may be the process that causes the damaging inflammation in the brain. In any case, we eat almost no added sugar. (We do get the sugar that's naturally occurring in fruits and in the *very* dark chocolate that is Michael's favorite treat.)

We avoid a lot of carbs because of gluten, but beyond that we make sure the carbs we do eat are nutritious and include fiber. In other words, no "white" carbs—white bread, white pasta, white rice, even white potatoes. When shopping for gluten-free items, be sure to read the label: just because it's gluten-free doesn't mean it's good for you. For example, some food manufacturers add sugar when they remove gluten. As with everything, it's not about just blindly following a rule. You have to understand your body and what goes into it. One last point: for us, gluten-free became a lot easier when we discovered a particularly good gluten-free spirit. So occasionally I propose a toast with Tito's vodka.

We are also careful about dairy and have removed cow's milk from our diet. We don't even miss it in our coffee, since almond milk is such a good substitute. Cheese is high in fat, and that fat is saturated, so we've mostly booted that as well, just as the MIND diet suggests. But the Mediterranean diet makes room for some cheese and yogurt, both of which we enjoy. We like goat cheese once in a while too, or ricotta or fresh mozzarella. Greek yogurt is also a good choice. Michael takes his with brain-boosting raw honey. But sometimes we use dairy-free yogurt, like Silk, instead.

What to Drink

Water should be your go-to drink. First, if you are drinking water, you are *not* drinking something sugary or otherwise full of unnatural substances (like our previous habit, Diet Coke). Drinking plenty of water brings a direct benefit as well: the brain needs to be fully hydrated to perform its best in a number of areas, including focus and memory. Being dehydrated can cause confusion.

The latest thinking on water is that there's no need for every person to get some specific amount of it every day (forget about eight glasses a day as a blanket rule). So I figure as long as we're drinking water several times a day, we're doing well. It's best to avoid reaching that point when you're truly thirsty—that goes for your loved one *and* for you.

I choose purified bottled water because I don't have room in my life to be worrying about what, exactly, is in the water coming out of my tap. Tap or bottled—you just want to get your water from a trusted source.

We always have lemons in the house, too, because a slice or a squeeze really perks up a glass of water. Bottled lemon juice also works if that's easier for you.

Tea is another great choice. Its main ingredient (by volume, anyway) is water, of course, and tea is full of powerful antioxidants. Tea contains one of the two most common types of antioxidants known as catechins, which are noted for promoting healthy blood flow, especially to the brain. (The other prime source of catechins is cocoa.)

Another brain booster in tea is the caffeine, which enhances focus, mood, and memory. It's a temporary boost, of course, but why not? Teas vary in the amount of caffeine they contain. A cup of black tea has, very roughly, twice as much caffeine as a cup of green (and less than half as much as a cup of coffee). Green tea is low enough in caffeine that most people don't have to worry about how much they drink or at what time of day. However, if you are particularly sensitive to caffeine, you might want to monitor your reactions to adding green tea to your life and adjust as necessary.

You get all the goodness of tea whether it is hot or iced. Either way, the key is that you have to brew it yourself. Dried mixes or bottled versions lose most of the naturally occurring nutrients, and a lot of them have added junk besides. If you like sweet tea, try using stevia so your healthful beverage does not come with a side of unhealthful sugar. We drink our hot tea the British way, substituting almond milk for the dairy version.

Aside from our morning coffee and red wine with dinner, we drink water and iced green tea throughout the day. For Michael, this may have been as much of a challenge as changing his diet overall, since he was never much of a water drinker before. But mostly it's just a matter of getting used to a new habit. Now, reaching frequently for a glass of water is a perfectly natural part of our new normal.

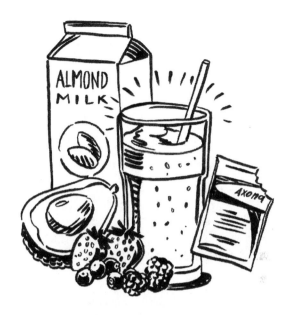

Caffeine and Medicine Don't Mix

While we're on the subject of what to drink, here's your coffee caveat: caffeine can interfere with the effect of some medicines used by Alzheimer's patients. So check with your doctor before you decide what's best. In our case, green tea doesn't contain enough caffeine to worry about, but we did learn not to mix it with his medicines. You don't have to cut out coffee altogether, but you may need to adjust the timing, as we did, or switch to decaf.

Go Organic

I'd been trying to eat healthy myself for many years by the time Michael was diagnosed. But eating organic was never part of the equation for me until I started looking into the best eating strategies for brain health. The more I read, the more I realized the importance of eating organic. Organic farming practices reduce pollution in the environment and our bodies. Plus, organic foods have a higher nutritional value compared to conventional food. So now I buy organic whenever possible. Eating organic has an unfairly bad rap as being expensive, but with a little bit of smart shopping I've kept my weekly grocery bill at about the same amount as before.

- Buy generic. I often buy generic brands instead of private labels, and that includes organic items. Almond butter is almond butter, especially those that contain only organic almonds and salt. Often, the generics are actually made by the exact same companies that supply the big brands anyway.
- Buy in bulk. If you really do go through a lot of something, buying in bulk can be significantly cheaper. For example, we buy big bags of frozen (organic) berries for smoothies, sacks of (organic) raw almonds big enough to last us six weeks, giant bottles of omega-3 supplements, and organic free-range, low-sodium chicken broth by the case. Michael and I love to shop together, and Costco or Sam's Club is a regular stop for us.
- Plan. Buy only what you need, especially when it comes to fresh food, so that it doesn't go to waste. Sometimes it happens, of course, but you want to avoid laying out money for fancy but delicate greens and then have them go to mush in your crisper before you get around to serving them. Make menus before you go shopping, keep on hand common ingredients that don't spoil quickly, and make quick trips to the market for fresh produce and seafood two or three times a week.

- Shop at a farmer's market. The lovely fruits and vegetables at a farmer's market are not only fresher and therefore longer lasting, but they also are much cheaper than they would be at the grocery or natural foods store.

Shopping at the farmer's market also helps me prioritize fresh foods in our eating plan. I avoid packaged foods and anything with preservatives whenever I shop. At the farmer's market, of course, that's incredibly easy to do since the stuff I'm trying to avoid isn't there anyway. You also might consider buying organic frozen fruits and vegetables if you cannot make frequent trips to the grocery store or a farmer's market. This gives you the option of including the best quality foods in your recipes.

When it comes to meat and fish, I go beyond organic and buy only grass-fed or wild-caught, again for the heart-healthy omega-3 fatty acids. Each filet may cost more than I used to pay, but we're rarely eating beef, so the costs seem to average out. Buying healthy fish is nonnegotiable, since including it in Michael's diet is "doctor's orders."

Medicine and Food

Many Alzheimer's medications go down easier with food rather than on an empty stomach. One of Michael's medications comes in a powdered form, which I can mix into a smoothie or other drink. We've also had luck minimizing side effects by having him take medication with a little Greek yogurt or oatmeal at breakfast. Morning works best for us and our medications, but talk to your doctor and then work out what's right for you.

Moderation

You can eat mostly anything you like if you eat everything in reasonable amounts. (And choose a lot of healthy foods, of course.) Some people are naturally better at portion control than others, so if it isn't clear how much of a food is good for you and how much is too much, you might want to study up on the subject. For me it's habit by now, but as I was starting out I learned a lot from Autumn Calabrese's *21 Day Fix* and *FIXATE* books.

Here are some simple, time-saving strategies I use to help keep us on track:

- Treat yourself. Following the MIND diet allows you to eat a wide range of foods. If your favorites are on the "limit" list, don't forget to build some of them into your eating plan. Go ahead and have prime rib or a thick, juicy burger, but infrequently. Love pie? Have a slice—sometimes. The trick is moderation. It is also important to embrace the idea that this is really a treat, not necessarily rare but really special. Savor it. With this attitude, you're likely to enjoy that burger even more than before.
- Share. Want a nice steak? Split it. Like a taste of something sweet at the end of a restaurant dinner? Order one dessert for the table along with several forks. Or share with yourself: at the beginning of a meal, set aside enough "leftovers" for lunch the next day before you even begin to eat. We love leftovers!
- Cook for yourself. We love to go out to eat, but most often I cook for us, usually with Michael as assistant chef. That way, I'm in control of what goes into what we eat. For example, I

can make sure there's no added sugar, use only half the salt called for, or substitute olive oil for butter. MIND has us avoiding fried foods. This means we grill a lot! But you also want to watch out for sauces and any other places sugar or saturated fats could be hiding.

Enjoy Your Meals

Mealtime is important to living well with Alzheimer's and not just because of the foods you are eating.

A meal is a social occasion, and that interaction is key for anyone dealing with Alzheimer's. Michael and I always eat together, and we often eat with others. When my kids are home, it's a family dinner. Going out with friends is still one of our favorite social activities. Even just the two of you eating together is a bonding experience. Dine leisurely. Enjoy your food. Unwind with a glass of red wine. Talk, even if it's about nothing in particular. This is not the time to complain about your situation or discuss whatever your accountant just pointed out.

Routine is also important to a person with Alzheimer's, and meals offer several ways to build structure into your day. It marks time, for example. Make sure eating is an activity that occurs in a predictable way each day.

Purposeful activity is another crucial component of maintaining function for as long as possible, and meal prep and cleanup are rife with opportunities for this kind of movement. Michael and I work together to handle duties for most meals. He usually helps me chop ingredients, set and clear the table, and run the dishwasher. I'm usually the one to cook. Even if one of us is just sitting there keeping the other company, it's still teamwork.

Tips and Tricks

- Don't stock what's not good for you. If you have it in the house, you'll eat it. Surround yourself with optimal choices instead.
- "Cheat." If someone else orders dessert and offers you a bite, take it. When your host offers something not on your usual menu, go ahead and sample. Life is short. Enjoy what you enjoy.
- How you think about your food matters. I try to stay away from a diet mentality—diets are hard and temporary. The way we're eating is really a long-term lifestyle choice. It's just how we roll.
- Don't take things away; just make healthy substitutions. You can substitute ground chicken or turkey for ground beef in your meatballs, for example, or brown rice pasta (gluten-free) for the wheat version. You'll get used to these types of changes quickly, and soon you won't miss whatever you swapped out. Even my kids don't complain about the brown pasta on their plates as long as it is topped with red sauce and (turkey) meatballs.
- Choose low-fat when you are eating foods that have saturated fats. Sometimes this means types of food that are naturally lower in fat, like goat cheese rather than brie, which has considerably more. Or select a lower fat version, like two-percent-fat yogurt, which is my go-to (the fat-free may sound tempting, but usually contains a lot of other gunk). Try to select white-meat chicken over dark every time: less fat in breast meat means less saturated fat in you. But you still get to enjoy a chicken dinner.
- Sprouted bread is a good gluten-free option, and brings with it a little extra nutrition. It's especially good toasted. Ezekiel

is one common brand, though you might have to look for it in the freezer section.
- For devoted carnivores, try pork tenderloin. It's very lean, and more heart healthy than a lot of beef, but meaty nonetheless. The same goes for veal.
- Eggs are a reasonable source of protein consistent with the MIND diet. Like all animal products, they contain saturated fat, which you are trying to limit, but overall they are very low in fat. Still, we each eat eggs only in moderation, maybe two or three times per week, because of Michael's cholesterol. When we do, we choose organic, of course, and pasture-raised (sometimes called "grass-fed"), because they are naturally higher in omega-3s (as well as other nutrients). You can also get "omega-3 eggs" from chickens that are given supplementary omega-3, with up to 200 mg of good omegas per egg. These are not usually organic, but on the other hand it's good to get as much omega-3 from food (as opposed to supplements) as possible.
- Sushi is one of our favorite ways to enjoy fish, and we make it an all-around healthy choice by getting it with brown rice.
- Eat dessert, but choose fruit, especially berries.
- Ask yourself: would this taste good with a little cinnamon? Most things do, so try to sprinkle it on everything you can think of. Cinnamon is good for blood sugar levels, and that's good for the brain. And how about a sprinkle of cocoa powder too? It's full of flavonol antioxidants.
- Not all olive oil is created equal. Use only extra virgin.
- Try almond milk. It's really good in coffee. This way, you're avoiding the inflammatory nature of dairy products but also

bringing the nutrition of the good fats in nuts to the table (or your coffee cup).
- You can hide a lot in a smoothie. Not that fond of kale? Overdosing on almonds? Add a bit of whatever you know is good for you (but don't love on its own) to a blender, and you have a healthy drink. I often put pomegranate seeds in smoothies because I love a dose of their resveratrol, which breaks down brain plaques. We love pomegranate, but there are only so many seeds you can eat at a given time. A smoothie is a great way to get more of them.
- Flax seeds are a good source of omega-3s, but it's not always obvious how to add them to your diet. My favorite way is in smoothies, but you also can stir them into yogurt or oatmeal, or sprinkle them on a salad.
- Snacks are powerful. Keep on hand and easily accessible (i.e. already prepared or portioned) healthy snack foods. Healthy snacks are great way to get MIND foods into your day. Frequent choices for us include a piece of fruit and a handful of nuts or raw veggies with hummus or nut butter.
- Use lots of herbs and you won't need much salt. Use sea salt when you really want it, but otherwise get your flavor boost from lemon juice, Dijon mustard, fresh ground black pepper, hot sauce, spices, and fresh herbs when possible.
- Chicken broth is your friend. It's easy to make yourself, but even easier to buy, as long as you find low-sodium and organic/free-range options. Adding chicken broth to your food is a great way to boost flavor and variety to fresh foods while keeping preparation easy. Toss steamed veggies with

a couple tablespoons of broth and use it instead of water to cook brown rice or quinoa.
- Decide what's for dinner together. Maintaining engagement with food choices is good for a lot of reasons. We always have fresh veggies with dinner, for example, but I'll ask Michael which of the available choices he's in the mood for. Or I'll ask if I should make chicken or fish and how he wants it prepared—with tomato and herbs, or lemon and olive oil? We also love to grocery shop together.
- Order together. When you're out to eat, healthful choices may not be first on anyone's mind. Besides, menus can be overwhelming, with too many choices. Or a person may simply forget what they really like. To avoid frustration, embarrassment, unnecessary "bad" stuff, or unwanted plates of food, suggest a couple choices for the two of you to split. You may say something like, "What do you think, the fish with the pistachio crust, or the Greek salad with chicken?"
- Embrace change together. Be patient with—but insistent upon—the transition you're making toward the healthiest way of eating.

I know this is a lot of information at once, but remember that you don't have to change everything tomorrow to make this work. The important thing is to get started. Make a change. Choose what works for you, in your life, for your body. Then make another choice. You'll get there!

As the Italians might say when raising a wine glass, *Salute!* To your health.

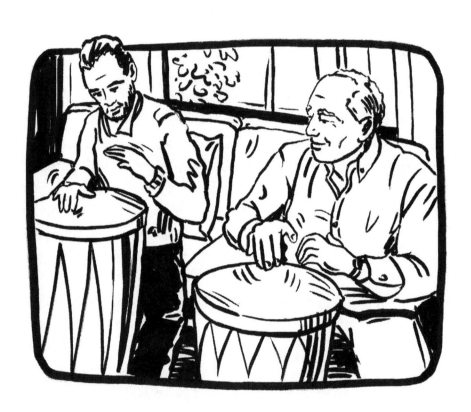

CHAPTER 4

BE CREATIVE

After Michael's diagnosis, I was a woman on a mission, looking for anything and everything that would stimulate his brain. I discovered over and over again the solid benefits—social, emotional, and cognitive—of engaging in creative activity of all kinds. Getting creative boosts self-esteem, releases stress and frustration, and allows self-expression even as a patient's skills diminish. Engaging in an artistic activity, in whatever form, facilitates communication, socialization, and various physical skills. It also tends to give you an experience of really being in the moment. Engaging creatively promotes positive feelings in general. Making something new (literally *creating*) is just a pleasurable experience, plain and simple, and that's never more true than it is for someone dealing with Alzheimer's, who often feels a profound sense of loss with regard to accomplishing daily activities. Being creative helps that loss become more manageable.

Music

With all this in mind, I wasted no time in signing Michael up for music lessons. I didn't need the scientific proof that music is powerfully therapeutic for people with Alzheimer's, though a body of evidence does in fact exist. Michael has loved music his whole life, both listening to and making it, so it was natural for him to pick it back up again.

Now his drumming lesson is a highlight of the week. I stay out of the way—this is guy time—but I hear Michael and his teacher jamming away together, with Michael chattering on, something he rarely does these days. I think getting back into familiar rhythms reminds him of his "garage band" days as a young man on the Jersey Shore. Michael was and is a mean drummer. And how many of us don't love a trip back to when we were at our coolest?

After each lesson/jam session, Michael is totally charged up and engaged for the rest of the day, like he had a Red Bull or something, with a definite gleam in his eye. The effect lasts for a long time and underscores the stimulating and fun part of music.

Noah Plotkin, Founder, Music Director, and CEO, LifeRhythmsInc.com

The part of the brain that stores music, melody, rhythm, and sound is pretty much the last one to be affected by Alzheimer's. Short-term memory may be shot, language skills might have faded, but music remains a strong way to communicate and connect. This goes double for those who played an instrument—those skills cling tenaciously in long-term memory. Most people can recall and sing song lyrics once you get them started—even people who can no longer speak. All this means that music remains a great way to engage a person for a long time, even as the disease progresses.

Making music or rhythms together results in a rich social experience. Percussion in particular adds a physical coordination challenge. Personally I think there's something else special about drumming. It produces vibrations you can feel, and so can the people around you. It's always a shared experience.

Each week, Michael and I do some stuff that is very familiar, but also some new stuff. We do the same warm-up exercises each time, for example—and, remarkably, he always remembers the patterns. Every week we also add something new, like putting a tambourine in the mix, or singing while also drumming. Sometimes it's familiar and new at the same time—like a beat we haven't done together before but is stored away in Michael's past experience. Recently, he drummed out a perfect bossa nova as soon as I got the groove started. Drawing on strengths while also providing new challenges is important.

Art

I've learned so much on this journey through Alzheimer's, and among the most surprising things is that *I* love art class! Sure, Michael is enjoying and reaping the benefits, but I am always ready to participate—anything that will make the experience richer and more enjoyable for Michael. Indeed, I'm getting as much out of it as he is. (Caregivers need as many opportunities as possible to build our inner resources.) I'd never taken an art class in my life; up to now my basic idea of a relaxing morning was a long cardio class. But from the very first day in Carole Pearlman's "The Art of Play," I was hooked. Those two and a half hours each week just fly by.

I got my first clue back when I watched Michael's initial art experience with our friend Jonathan, who agreed to teach him doodling and drawing with watercolors and watercolor crayons. Jonathan left a bunch of supplies at our house, leaving me with specific instructions to make art in ways that would be meaningful for us together. It should be, he said, a joint experience. I had to get over my "but I'm no artist" attitude. In this case, Michael became *my* role model, because he is never judgmental about what he makes; he just goes for it. When he creates something, he is completely in the moment.

Now both Michael and I get totally engaged with class projects. Engagement is the name of the game for someone with Alzheimer's, so this is definitely a "win." I also appreciate anything that simply fills a significant chunk of time but in a meaningful way. Plus, the shared interest and activity help us stay connected. Having fun together will do that! It's new territory for both of us, and doing it together makes us both more motivated to give it a try.

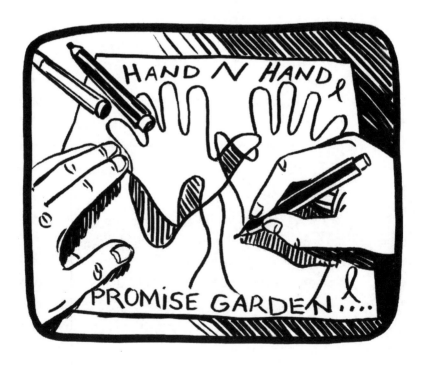

Jonathan Plotkin, Editorial Illustrator and Cartoonist; Spontoonist.com

I've been a friend of Michael's and Cheryl's for a long time—I knew him first in his days as a real estate executive. I'm an illustrator and cartoonist, not a licensed art therapist, and I don't have any training in Alzheimer's, but I am a big believer in the power of art as a transformative vehicle for people who would not otherwise be able to express themselves. Because making art is such a primal aspect of human beings, it is one of the last things to go even as memory fails.

My work with Michael was an experiment. I wanted to engage Michael, to help him open up a way to communicate, to express his individuality, and to find the joy in the process. The results were astonishing. He was immediately focused on that moment; nothing could distract him. He followed my lead easily and enthusiastically. I'd also use the opportunity to just talk with him, and he was able to be very verbally communicative while he was doing art. I'd use certain forms and images to try to pull remembrances out of him too. The time I drew a building, for instance, he immediately recognized as a Home Depot. I often teach how doodling helps the half of the population who are visual learners to remember things better. I can't say Michael was learning more with art—his disease imposes terrible limitations—but he was making connections that would otherwise have been fleeting. That's the power of art and imagery, and the pure joy of creating.

Dance

Our newest creative outlet is dance therapy. Michael and I have always loved to dance together whenever we get the opportunity, and especially to big band music. So when I saw the listing for a daytime class featuring big band music, I suddenly wondered why we hadn't done this before! In the end, we opted for lessons at home rather than the hubbub of a big group class. I was thrilled when I found Erica Hornthal, who is a licensed dance/movement therapist with a background in both dance and counseling. She teaches classes at the senior center, but came to the house a few times to work one on one with Michael and me. That was an excellent introduction and a way to get comfortable, while in the familiar surroundings of our home, with a new person and a new skill, so we just decided to keep going!

As a creative activity and a form of self-expression, stress-relief, and so on, dance comes with the additional benefit of being excellent physical exercise. Depending on how you do it, it can be a real workout, but even if you don't break much of a sweat you are practicing balance, coordination, and other skills that can enhance overall wellbeing. Partner dancing also fosters communication between two people, in addition to being just a nice bit of couple time. For us, it's an intimate connection. Plus, it's incredibly fun!

Mix It Up

For Michael, dancing, and dance therapy, is all about the music. In our case, dance class stimulates the brain by tapping into a longstanding interest—music—and by introducing new, enjoyable experiences.

Dancing combines music and movement, and we've had similar success combining music and art. In our art class, the teacher always plays music when we get down to work: it's a part of the experience both Michael and I love. I can see how the music changes Michael's whole approach—his strokes are freer, his colors more vivid, his creative juices obviously get flowing. I believe the combination helps different parts of the brain connect.

Okay, You Convinced Me—Where Do I Sign Up?

We use a lot of private lessons—though lately I've become a fan of the local parks-and-rec offerings. But it isn't necessary to hire your own teacher to get the benefits of creative activities. Every community has something to offer, though they won't necessarily invite you to join; you need to seek them out. Check out your local senior center, community center, rec center, and memory care center. A lot of school districts also run classes for adults in their buildings at night and on weekends. An online search will turn up many options—and so will a visit to that old-fashioned but ever-popular community bulletin board, like the ones in the post office and the coffee shop near me.

Most, if not all, of the classes you find should be much less expensive than having a teacher visit your home. Still, you need to choose the *right* class for your situation. The specifics of what makes it right may vary from person to person, but for us we've learned that 1) a small class is important—not too many names and faces, 2) personalized attention from the teacher is a must, and 3) it needs to be conveniently located. The instructors don't have to be specially trained in working with people with Alzheimer's, but they do have to welcome the challenge, practice inclusiveness in their teaching, and be willing to try new approaches as necessary. In most cases, you can get a lot of clues if you actually read the website, catalog entry, or flyer describing the class. Reading something about "Strengthening the right brain one art experience at a time" was what drew me to the art class we're enrolled in now. A description filled with jargon, or marked for "advanced beginners," told me that class wasn't for us.

The needs of a person with Alzheimer's may also vary over time. Michael first took a photography class following his diagnosis. And it was great—for a while. Eventually, the mechanics of working the camera become too complex for him. What had started as a stimulating experience eventually became frustrating and, hence, no longer helpful. So we moved on.

You might also want to keep in mind that for some people, at varying points, a class isn't as good a fit as one-on-one instruction. Generally, the interaction of a group setting is a benefit, but if it is overwhelming—too big, too loud, too confusing—it won't be a good choice. (Another thing about that photography class was that it had about 20 people in it, which ultimately became too overwhelming for Michael.)

Communicate

To give the teacher the best chance of making the class a good fit for you and your loved one, *communicate*. In advance. Call, send an email, or otherwise reach out to let the teacher know what to expect and how he or she can help. I always explain why I might be hanging around class—and why I might leave. I emphasize that my goal is for Michael to do as much as possible independently, but also to make sure he is comfortable and successful in whatever class he takes.

You'll work out some of the details on the fly. For instance, in an early art class the teacher asked Michael what color he wanted and, like I knew he would, Michael didn't answer. I knew he was paralyzed by that kind of open-ended question. I asked if he wanted pink, green, or blue, and then he made his choice. I've learned that choosing among a small number of specific options like that is always easier for someone with Alzheimer's. Later I followed up with the teacher about this exchange and—hallmark of a good teacher—she said she'd noticed the difference in approach and intended to adopt it.

In general, you want to determine if the teacher has any experience with special needs in general or Alzheimer's in particular. It doesn't have to be official training. Some of Michael's teachers who have brought the best insight to the process simply have a loved one with the disease or an open, curious, and problem-solving mind. You want to get a sense of whether the person will be sensitive to and comfortable with a person with Alzheimer's. There's no checklist for figuring this out, but I've discovered a lot about how an instructor will handle the situation by the way he or she responds to my questions and concerns.

Do It Yourself

Of course, you don't necessarily need any class or teacher at all to get into creative activities. Since we had so much fun in art class, we went out and stocked up on supplies to keep at our house—oil crayons, water colors, paper, and so on. Some other things we've enjoyed at home, though they are too "unofficial" for class, are coloring books (the ones designed for adults—no need to be coloring characters from the movie *Frozen*) and paint-by-numbers sets (less than ten dollars at the toy store). I always put on music when we get down to work on an art project, so we just tap into all kinds of creative energy. We like to do it with a fire going in the fireplace and a glass of wine at hand. We often take our inspiration from what we've experienced in class, but you can search online for cool projects and techniques, and try whatever appeals to you.

You can do music at home too—everything from listening to favorites (around here, that's Jimmy Buffet) and singing or tapping along to playing your own instruments. And if a little dancing breaks out, so much the better! For an easy way to fill your home with music, check out the music channel options from your cable provider. We have one on almost all the time, unless of course we're watching a show.

You can even learn to drum without any previous experience. I'd suggest getting yourself a little guidance (YouTube has *everything*) to get the most out of it—though even two people just making noise banging on pots and pans can be fun, cathartic, and interactive. With a little more knowhow, though, you can make the most of the more grounding effects of drumming together.

Anyone can get creative; no experience is necessary. The process is what matters most. The finished product is a bonus (and something you can display at home!). Just keep in mind that the process is the point, and is way, way more important than the finished product. No need for you to be Astaire, Picasso, or Sinatra to have a great time, connect with yourself and others, and stimulate your brain.

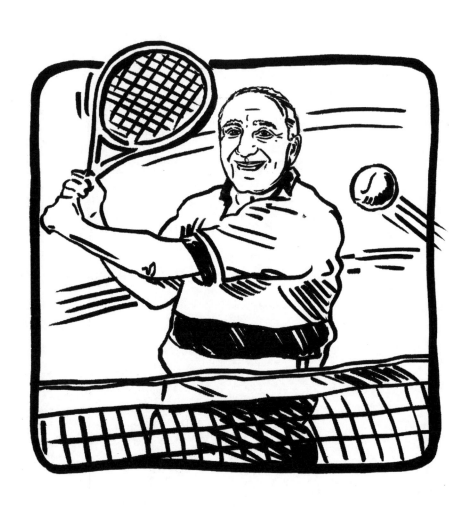

CHAPTER 5

FINDING A "BUDDY"

About three times a week for three or four hours, Michael goes out with his buddy, Lee. They go golfing, bowling, or maybe to a movie. Sometimes they get a beer and play cards. On some days, they go to the gym or play tennis. They talk stocks. They reminisce about their pre-retirement careers.

They do guy stuff.

And then Lee collects a paycheck. He's a professional caregiver. And his decision to give back to the community in this way, in his retirement, has been an unbelievable gift to Michael and me. I'm beyond grateful for his work and for Matt Field, owner of a home healthcare agency, who first let me know this kind of care was even an option. Where my image of a home caregiver was a lady in scrubs maneuvering someone in a wheelchair, Matt helped me see a wider range of options. Most people don't "see" this kind of caregiver out in the world, mostly because Lee and Michael just look like two friends out for the day.

The Buddy System

If I were the patient, and I needed a buddy, we would probably engage in different activities, like mah-jongg or pottery class or some kind of girls'-night-out stuff. But for Michael, I think the male friendship is particularly important in this equation. After his diagnosis, some of our friends drew closer, but some pulled away, particularly the men. (See Chapter 13: Be Interactive for some strategies to keep friendships going successfully.) Even those who didn't pull back are about Michael's age and not retired. So they are not around during the day for a game of golf or tennis, or biking, or whatever hobby they enjoy. That's why it's been especially fulfilling for Michael to have that male camaraderie with Lee. They have become true friends.

It's also great for Michael to have regular—and positive—interaction with someone, anyone, other than me. It's obviously good for me—I get a little time in my day to deal with the rest of life, including taking care of myself, while knowing he's in great hands. It's also important for each of us to have our personal time, like any couple, but even more so now. For Michael, knowing he can be out and about without me is a key piece of maintaining as much independence as possible. His interactions with Lee, and the world he goes out into with Lee, are empowering.

Their outing also gives Michael something concrete to look forward to. It's always a positive experience, something enjoyable. For Michael, it is an excellent anchor to his routine. When he doesn't have 'Lee time' (even Lee needs some time off), it throws Michael off a little. He's just not as focused when his routine is altered, so it's important to prepare for those times when Lee will be away.

"I Don't Need Help"

This whole subject can be a really tough sell; I'm not going to lie. Hiring someone to help out is a symbol of diminishing abilities that nobody looks forward to. Maybe you need someone with nursing skills or help with bathing.

Having a conversation about a "buddy" may be easier than discussing the possibility of hiring a "caregiver" or even "companion." For example, people who have had to give up driving might like to know that a buddy could 'chauffeur' them around town. You might focus on the fact that having a buddy can mean *not* having to give up hobbies you enjoy. Once our conversations began to focus on a way for Michael to hang out and enjoy activities in his retirement (our search began when I was still working full time), Michael became more open to the possibility. For some people, the idea of having a "personal assistant" might be more appealing—and more fitting in some circumstances anyway, depending on the activities involved.

One more strategy that might be useful is talking to the person with Alzheimer's about how accepting outside help helps *you*. Of course this depends on the stage of the disease, but for some people, thinking of getting help as a way *they* can take care of *you* can make a big difference in their perspective and add a different, more positive meaning to the experience. In other words, if your loved one with Alzheimer's understands that getting help is as much about you as it is about him or her, you might notice a shift in attitude.

It's important for everyone to share their feelings about getting extra help; it needs to be a joint decision, with everyone on board. Enter the 24-Hour Rule—neither of us had to like the idea of hiring help, but we didn't keep griping about it either. We talked about it—what bothered us about the prospect of bringing a stranger into our home and lives, and the pros and cons. Then we *moved on*. We found Matt and then he introduced us to Lee.

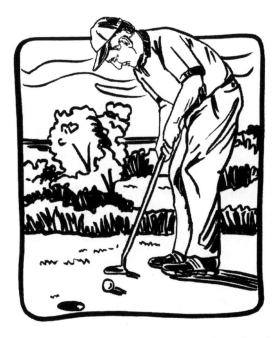

Once we hired Lee, I treated his visits as if Michael were meeting with a friend. Happily, with one round of golf, Michael and Lee hit it off immediately. That Lee is a great golfer is a bonus! Now, Lee is a highly anticipated part of Michael's regular routine.

Matt Field, Owner and Operator, Right at Home
Matt Field of Right at Home helped us find Lee. The company's mission, he explained, is to provide physical, emotional, and cognitive support to a person with Alzheimer's. "We want to increase wellness, keep people active physically and cognitively, and delay progression as much as possible," he says. For Michael, this would mean a person who could make sure he was safe, yes, but more importantly keep him active, socializing, independent, and engaged with the world. I was on board!

Still, when I asked Matt why it's important to get help in the home for a person with Alzheimer's, he first said that getting outside helps increase family caregiver wellness. In other words, I should get someone to work with Michael because it would help me. And I do realize now how much Michael's time with Lee means to me. I go the gym, play tennis (working out has always been my major source of stress relief), or go play mah-jongg. Retirement is new for me, so I'm still learning what it means to really take care of myself in this situation, but I know enough to say that these protected times in my schedule are critical to the whole process. (See Chapter 10: Care for the Caregiver for more on this topic.)

Also, right at the top of Matt's list of things to know about hiring caregivers is to call before you need the help so that you avoid the burnout that arises from caregiving solo. Even if you don't plan to hire right now, call around anyway—don't wait—to learn about your options. Find an agency you feel comfortable with. Then store all that information away safely somewhere so that when you do need it you'll be ready to roll. I simply said to Michael, "I know we don't need this yet, but let's look into it so we'll be ready when you do." It's never too soon to start, Matt assures me. In fact, if he had his way, every family would be familiar with a home care agency so when a need arises they have one fewer decision to make. Anyone could break a leg or get sick, and need some help for a while, so it's best to be prepared.

How to Find Your "Lee"

Although you can't have our Lee, rest assured that you *can* find someone like him. When you contact an agency for help hiring a companion, ask if there are people like this on their roster. Not everyone will offer this kind of buddy system. Services have challenges finding individuals who want to act in this role. Lee, for example, was looking for volunteer opportunities when he first met Matt. (And he did volunteer for years at a rehab and memory care center, where he helped family members learn how to support their loved ones.) But Matt was the one to ask Lee if he'd be interested in this kind of role.

More than ever, the caregiver role is changing, especially for early-onset Alzheimer's and early-stage Alzheimer's, and it's a big change for the better. But this change—including this "buddy" model—is occurring too slowly. You may have to be the one to educate service providers on what you believe is important, because you are the best advocate for your loved one with Alzheimer's. In this case, your job comes with a bonus: when you succeed in getting a service to find you a buddy, you're clearing the path for others who are walking with you. You might have to talk someone into recruiting a "buddy," and, later, they might suggest the same to someone who doesn't know to ask for it. It's a win-win.

I can't promise it will be *easy* to find your own Lee, but it can be done. If services don't come through for you, try hiring on your own. Word of mouth is almost always your best bet. However, you might not get personal referrals specific to a "buddy" since it's a fairly new category of caregiver. Try colleges and even medical and other health-care schools with job boards that make it easy to reach out to the students. Students studying pre-med, psychology, gerontology, or some other relevant field have flexible schedules and youthful energy. Plus, they often need money and job experience. If you hire someone on your own, you may have more flexibility with scheduling, and you will probably save some money compared to working with an agency. But then you will be responsible for all employee-related issues. With an agency, you know the caregivers have been fully vetted and trained. Plus, going through an agency means you have access to a Plan B if something doesn't work out with a particular caregiver, like a sick day, which can throw everyone's schedule off.

As you begin your search, look for someone who's generally patient, personable, and pleasant to be with. It's much easier to find a buddy who already possesses these characteristics (versus attempting to train someone to become the kind of companion who will enhance your loved one's daily life). And if you can find an individual with experience conversing with a person with Alzheimer's, all the better.

For me, it was important to find a person who would engage Michael, not simply park him in front of the television. You may have observed caregivers like that—reading the paper at a restaurant instead of talking with their clients. But the interaction—the socializing—is key. You need someone to provide loving care, of course, with deep reserves of patience. Look for someone who accepts this illness for what it is and doesn't deny it, get scared by it, or overly cater to it.

Also, you want someone who is extremely even-keeled and, ideally, someone who shares the same interests as your loved one. That way the two of them have a foundation for building a real relationship. If you're lucky, what you'll find is someone who simply has a 'knack' for caregiving—a "buddy natural."

You'll also want to consider selecting someone who can help you with specific tasks. Ask yourself, for example, "Do I need someone who can drive?" "Does this person need his or her own car?" In our case, we needed someone eager to be active, who loved sports, and who could talk intelligently about business. Michael was not going to be happy with someone who wasn't athletic or who didn't have the ability to follow the stock market, something he's always enjoyed.

What you *don't* need is an Alzheimer's expert. (If you find one, and he or she meets all your other requirements, that's okay too.) As long as someone is willing to learn and to learn from experience, it should be fine. The other qualities are more important than specific Alzheimer's knowledge.

Your goal is to find the right person for you and your loved one—the right skills, attitude, and experience for what is needed now. As time goes on, your needs will change, and you can add a different caregiver if that becomes necessary. Transitions are not easy, but sometimes they're necessary, especially as the disease progresses.

Mr. Wrong

If you hire the wrong person, you'll know it. But that's okay; once you know, do something about it. When I was still working, we needed additional help during the winters while Michael was in Florida. The person we hired "babied" Michael and that didn't work for us at all. Michael didn't want to stay with him for even a short while. Plus, I thought he would create too much dependency in Michael. We even had Lee train this person, but he just didn't really "get" the mindset of empowering Michael. So we moved on.

Buddy Management

If you enlist family and friends as buddies, they will need help and encouragement. Providing detailed instructions that include suggested activities and communication strategies will make their time with your loved one more productive.

Even professionals may need similar support, especially if they haven't been in the "buddy" role before. You may well be asking for something a bit different from what they learned in any training they received. In any case, you have to be very clear about what you want—and what you *don't* want—out of the pairing.

Everyone will need encouragement, not just to find the best activities but also to walk the line between pretending nothing is wrong and treating a person with Alzheimer's as if he or she is completely helpless. In that center lane is where a buddy will be able to provide the support necessary to help the person with Alzheimer's be as independent and successful as possible.

For example, I insisted any buddy for Michael wear regular clothes, not any kind of uniform. No scrubs, no polo with company logo, no carrying a clipboard wherever they go. I wanted Michael and his buddy to do what friends do, and while they were doing it I wanted them to look no different from any other two guys going out for a beer or whatever. This was more than just a superficial concern; it helped Michael accept the relationship. The relationship provides an interactive, social experience for Michael—his buddy is not a babysitter.

You will probably want to be the one to select the activities for your loved one and buddy, at least at first. Lee and I connect via text the night before an outing, and I suggest a few activities I think will work for Michael and his schedule. I try to alternate their activities, so that Michael always has a variety of things to do. If there's a task I think Michael needs practice with, or one I think he needs to avoid (temporarily or otherwise), I'll suggest activities accordingly. Lee knows by now what Michael enjoys—what they enjoy together—so he always has good ideas. But he doesn't live with Michael like I do, so he can't know all the ins and outs of Michael's current status. I always check in to get feedback from Lee as well.

Hiring the right person is an important first step, but from there developing a good working relationship is paramount.

Meet Lee Gimbel, Michael's Buddy

I've got no special cure for Michael. I just respect him, listen to him, try to make him happy. I aim to be kind, like I would be to anybody. I always treat everyone how I would like to be treated—with respect. That worked all through my long career in the business world, way back when I had a job at a therapeutic school. This essential approach works with my other friends and, of course, with Michael.

A caregiver does have to have certain qualities. I'm patient—you have to be for this line of work. And I'm caring, which is right there in the name: care-giver. And that's it. Those are the things that are most important.

Michael and I have been meeting for more than three years now, and from my perspective he's going through this very well. He has not regressed a lot over time, not in real obvious ways, at least. He enjoys being social. He likes to talk over all the places he traveled for his career, and about his trips to Florida.

Sometimes he forgets items he brought with him, but that's no big deal. Sometimes he forgets how to finish a sentence once he's started, but I just fill in or change the subject. I try to be encouraging, and reinforce all the things that he does well.

He's a really active guy, and so that's most of what we do together—taking a walk, playing bocce or tennis. He goes all out at the gym, and I don't think he cares that I am ten years older than he is and it isn't always easy to keep up! Do all the crossword puzzles you want, but I think exercise is really the best possible thing. It aerates your brain.

Help! You Need Somebody

Whether you and your loved one are in need of a buddy or someone with more specific skills, the important thing is to recognize that you, indeed, need help—and what kind you really need and want. Accepting help is a challenge for many people with Alzheimer's, and perhaps an even greater challenge for their family caregivers. But don't let this particular challenge stop you. You have the skills, and I hope I've given you a set of tools to help you find a buddy who's the right fit for your loved one.

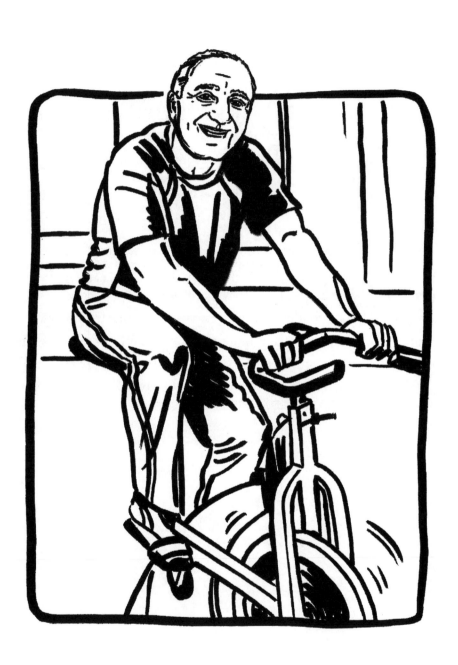

CHAPTER 6

EXERCISE FOR MIND AND BODY

Okay, here's a piece of the puzzle that may be a tough change: get more exercise. Maybe a *lot* more exercise. Anyone who knows us can tell you: Michael and I are exercise nuts. When my friends call my cell, they don't ask where I am; they just say, "You at the club?" Biking, hiking, tennis—the list goes on. Michael and I have spent a lot of time doing this kind of stuff together for as long as we've been a couple. Since Michael's diagnosis, we've become more focused in our approach to exercise as an important part of our quest for the brain-healthiest way of life possible. I'm convinced it's a major part of how Michael has maintained status quo for as long as he has.

You don't need to go to the same lengths we have to get the brain benefits of exercise. You should probably be moving every day, with enough effort that you get at least a little bit sweaty, but not so much that it feels hard or stressful. Our internist, Dr. Lee Freedman, calls that "moderate exercise"—you're working hard, but you should still be able to carry on a conversation. For most workouts for non-exercise fanatics, that's what you're aiming for. And you should *enjoy* exercise. It should feel good.

Anyone can do it, even a member of our national couch-potato club. Get up and take a walk outside. Sign up for a class at your rec center. Or try that elliptical set up in front of the TV in your friend's basement. Go play basketball or catch with your son/daughter (borrow someone else's if you need to!). Don't worry about making it perfect; just get moving. Solid research backs up the fact that even something you might consider a hobby and not *exercise* can give you the benefits of a body in motion, like gardening or going dancing (or just dancing around your living room), as long as you do it regularly.

Exercise is crucial for optimal brain function. As I dug into the topic of exercise and Alzheimer's, and what kind of exercise is best for the brain, I quickly found many sources explaining the ways heart health supported brain health. I also discovered that exercise improves circulation, which carries more oxygen to the brain. Exercise, over the long term, is one of the strongest protectors against Alzheimer's (though it's not a guarantee). One of my missions is to help everyone I know recognize that it's never too soon to start building up that benefit. Plus, it turns out that exercise is one of the best ways to tame Alzheimer's symptoms once they've begun, underscoring the notion that it's also never too late to begin. Exercise helps the brain and body preserve overall functioning at the highest level for the longest time possible.

Digging a little deeper, I learned a host of other reasons exercise is so helpful in maintaining a high quality of life with Alzheimer's, some of them quite surprising. With each additional benefit I discovered, I got more determined to make exercise a *big* part of our quest to make the most of our "new normal."

Soon we became more focused: we spent more time on exercise, we added in some new things, and we adjusted techniques to maximize brain benefit. We "officially" exercise *every single day*. After

Michael was diagnosed, we kept playing tennis like we always had (a few times a week when the weather allowed) and continued to bike, but Michael also began to join me in a year-round "cardio tennis" class. We took lessons to play paddle tennis too. Michael gets to play golf more often now than he did before he retired, at least once a week, though that too is dependent on the weather. And we stepped up our activity and time at the gym. We are there almost every single day for a combination of weights and cardio machines. Michael began working twice a week with Jason, a personal trainer at the gym. Jason customizes an optimal exercise program for him each time they meet.

We get a lot of "unofficial" exercise daily as well by walking, swimming, biking, taking a hike. We even signed up for a social dance class. I am convinced that keeping active has notably slowed the progression of the disease. Some of Michael's skills have actually increased, like coordination and functionality, and focus and attention. This, I am told, is highly unusual. Michael is definitely more interactive on days he exercises. If he misses a day for some reason, he is a lot less engaged, quieter. All this exercise has also helped Michael lose about 15 pounds, even as he's gaining muscle weight—he's trimmer now than he's been, perhaps, since he played college ball.

I've also experienced good results. I exercise with Michael to care for both of us mentally and physically. It's a great stress reducer, for sure. This is a long road, and for anyone taking care of a loved one, being healthy and happy yourself is vital to your ability to travel the journey.

Exercise doesn't have to be a thing that occurs during certain activities, or by following specific procedures, to be good for you.

There's no one "right" way to do it; what's right for you might change from day to day. The important thing is just to do it. As Jason says, "It's all about movement, sweat, and smiles." If you're moving your body, breaking a sweat, and having fun, you're doing it right.

Exercise Because ...

Following an Alzheimer's diagnosis, commit to exercise because it's good for your overall health, good for your heart health, and specifically good for your brain. Do it for all the reasons exercise is good for anyone:

- it lowers the risk of many chronic diseases;
- you'll get stronger muscles and stronger bones;
- it'll help you maintain a healthy weight;
- it improves your balance, your flexibility, and your eye-hand coordination;
- you'll look and feel better with regular exercise;
- it stimulates the release of feel-good endorphins in your body;
- it increases energy levels;
- it relieves stress; and
- it improves mood.

All these things take on an extra layer of importance for someone with Alzheimer's. For example, studies have linked obesity both with risk of Alzheimer's *and* faster progression of the disease. Many chronic diseases negatively impact brain function and/or risk of Alzheimer's. Alzheimer's affects the brain in various ways, among them impairing balance and eye-hand coordination. Exercise, on the other hand, lowers the risk of falls and injuries. Alzheimer's often saps self-confidence; looking and feeling better—common outcomes of exercise—builds it. Alzheimer's can cause low energy levels at the wrong time of day, and exercise counters that. Alzheimer's often comes with a side of depression and/or anxiety, both of which can be reduced by exercise.

Getting exercise was important before receiving the diagnosis. It's doubly important now. Care partners, this goes for you too. You are definitely going to need some of that stress-busting, endorphin-releasing goodness. Regular exercise is one of the best ways to protect a brain, to reduce the risk of Alzheimer's, and delay development of the disease's symptoms.

Strategies for Exercising with Alzheimer's

Like everything else in this new normal, your mantra for figuring out how best to exercise is going to be "patience and flexibility." Beyond that, I admit that the top two strategies for exercise for a person with Alzheimer's seem to be opposites. But don't let that stop you from getting the best of both worlds! Here they are:

1. Do whatever you already know how to do, what you have the most experience with, what is most familiar.
2. Learn something new.

Put another way: build on strengths; challenge weaker areas. With Alzheimer's, short-term memory declines before long term. The more you practice the former, the more support you give where it is needed most. The more you draw on the latter, the more successful you will be with whatever you undertake. And the more you reinforce that area of relative strength, the longer you will be able to draw on it.

Exercising in whatever way you've enjoyed most in your life should be a prominent part of what you do now. Even if this means reaching way into your past, your muscle memory will be there to support you. Been a regular attendee at yoga class for decades? Adjust as necessary, but there's no reason to step off the mat now. Old-fashioned bodybuilding or walking may help you connect to memories of your basic exercise program. Club tennis champ when you were young? Tennis drills might be your best bet now, even if you haven't really played in years. Grew up dancing? Formal or informal movement to music is probably just the thing now. This is the strategy Jason taps into when he lays an exercise ladder out on the gym floor. These days, Michael is struggling with "cross-body" movement—like the classic opposite-arm, opposite-leg pattern. But football footwork drills, like the ones they use tires for in the movies, the ones he spent many hours on in his school days? No problem! A kind of automatic pilot kicks in.

We're getting ready to add a new way to pursue the other angle to our repertoire: dance class! We've already used it by taking up paddle tennis. That one's actually a combination strategy: building on the familiar (tennis), but learning something new (paddle court). We do it for fun, to keep moving in ways we enjoy, and to have activities we share. But science backs up the benefit to the brain. For example, learning a new sport increases the size of the area of the brain related to movement control (the motor cortex) in the adult brain. This is a thing that until recently was generally thought to happen pretty much only through childhood! The growth does *not* happen by continuing to practice a skill that's already well honed. It's the process of picking up something new that builds the area.

Besides, learning something new just feels good. It's fun! (As long as you are reasonably patient with yourself.) There's no doubt Michael is energized by branching out in a new direction—he hates cold and snow as much as he loves to play sports, but paddle is a winter sport and it is played outside. The court you're standing on is heated, but the "walls" around you are only fencing! We play in our ski parkas.

With everything you do, it's important to find a balance that includes challenge but does not provoke stress. You never want frustration to outweigh fulfillment. You're going to be constantly pinging among "do what you can," "know your limits," and "keep trying." The key is to observe the person's reactions, and adjust as necessary. Like everything else about this journey through your new normal, you need to bring your patience, your flexibility, and your creative thinking as you navigate the road ahead.

How Does This Thing Work?

Perhaps the details don't matter to you—exercise has been shown to help, and that's good enough for you. Go ahead and just get moving! But for those who would like a little more insight, this section of the book is for you. I know it's long, but it's worth it!

Moving the body stimulates the brain, and it does this in a number of ways, all of which are good for brain function. Moving the body directly stimulates the brain by increasing oxygen flow to and in the brain, via the pumping of blood all around the body. This happens while you are actually exercising (so long as you do so enough to feel your heart rate increase at least a little bit)—that's why many people feel clearer in their minds for a while after exercise, Alzheimer's or not. Even more important, though, regular exercise, over time, increases blood flow to the brain in general (not just while you are working out). Oxygen is really, really important to the brain. The brain uses way more than its fair share (by weight) of all the oxygen in the body. The more oxygen that gets there via exercise, the better.

Furthermore, exercise releases chemicals that help the brain function better. And it reduces the amount of Alzheimer's notorious amyloid plaques in the brain. On top of all *that*, over time, physical activity actually increases the volume of the brain, creating new brain cells and perhaps even more blood vessels, and building more connections between cells and/or between parts of the brain. New cells are concentrated in areas of the brain most connected with learning and memory—at least in rats, which scientists have reason to believe match humans in this respect. Long-term exercise can also decrease the extent of the "holes" in brain tissue that Alzheimer's causes, and reduce the brain shrinkage associated with Alzheimer's.

Exercise also benefits the heart, and what's good for the heart is good for the brain. Many things that increase the risk of heart disease also increase the risk of dementia—smoking, for example, or high blood pressure. Things that protect the heart tend to protect the brain as well, like lowering cholesterol levels or controlling blood sugar levels. Or, perhaps most powerfully of all, exercise.

Dr. Chad Yucus, Neurologist
Physical exercise can help maintain motor function in spite of cognitive changes, which is what has happened in Michael's case. This is

an important part of staying active, functioning, and engaged with everyday life. The better a person's level of fitness, the better they'll usually do, and Michael is especially strong and active. But as long as you are maintaining a regular level of activity—even if it is less than what Michael accomplishes—you'll be getting the benefits.

Surprising Benefits of Exercise

For a person dealing with Alzheimer's symptoms, exercise offers a variety of other benefits that you might not immediately think of. I think these are just as important as the direct physical benefits, and they are a big part of why Michael has continued to function as long as he has at status quo.

Exercise can provide:

- Empowerment. Michael has long been a fan of bicycling, and because he now follows a well-established familiar route, he still goes on his own. For him, biking equals freedom.
- Independence. If it is feasible for a person to exercise on his or her own, that's a good thing to keep in rotation as long as it is possible/safe. In another sense of "independence," exercise improves strength, balance, and so forth, and therefore supports and develops the ability to manage other parts of one's life independently. This is "functionality"—the ability to keep doing everyday activities that take more physical coordination than we usually stop to think about, like brushing teeth, climbing the stairs, and loading the dishwasher. Preserving functionality is a huge part of living well with Alzheimer's.

- A sense of purpose. Participating in activities that have a clear point to them—exercise being one great example—is an important part of sustaining a high quality of life. Everyone likes to feel productive, pursue a passion, or set and accomplish a goal.
- Confidence. Continuing with activities you are good at—and/or learning new activities—builds confidence and provides motivation to continue. (You do have to be careful to avoid activities that cause only frustration.) For that matter, so does just looking and feeling good.
- Routine. Exercise is a way to connect with your "regular" self and the rest of your life up until the diagnosis.
- Feeling of competence and accomplishment. Alzheimer's often creates a feeling of helplessness, and exercise is one way to experience taking charge of the situation, and getting stuff done.
- Improved sleep. Alzheimer's can throw off the sleep-wake cycle, and exercise can curb that.
- A feel-good energy boost. You may be tired after a workout, but you also feel pretty jazzed. Your brain gets an instant buzz from exercise too, and it can be enough to decrease confusion or fogginess for a while.
- Routine. Especially for a person who has stopped working, maintaining a regular schedule is key—and a predictable time for exercise daily is one great way to give structure to the day.
- Brain stimulation. Anything that stimulates the brain is good for a person with Alzheimer's, but that does not only mean doing crosswords or playing music. Exercise stimulates the brain in various ways, all of them good, from sending it extra

oxygen to giving it practice following directions or using muscles in a new pattern to the mental challenge of keeping score or learning a new move. There's a lot of sensory stimulation with exercise too.

- Practice planning, organizing, direction-following, and goal-setting.
- A way to practice sustaining focus or attention. Some types of exercise work on this explicitly, like yoga or tai chi, but any type of activity that requires concentration can help.
- Social contact. This is a big one. Socializing is so important, but often difficult, for people with Alzheimer's. A social activity that does *not* focus on talking is often more comfortable and successful—hello, exercise! Exercise can be a social event—a good way to spend time with people—whether you take a class or get together for a hike with friends. Exercise is a good way to connect with people you already know, and a good way to interact with new people. Exercise can also provide opportunities to practice social skills, like when you are following directions in a class or with a trainer, or just interacting with a fellow exerciser.
- A chance to have fun! Working out may not always be fun, but it can be. Maybe sometimes it's simply pleasant. Or invigorating. But I think Michael enjoys physical exercise most when it is playful. Jason (the personal trainer) told me Michael is never happier in the gym than when he throws him a football. A game of catch wasn't exactly what I envisioned when as I signed up for our gym membership, but it meets one of Jason's key criteria for the best exercise: it makes Michael smile.

By the way, caregivers could do with a lot of these benefits too. Caregiving can be an isolating, stressful, emotional, and draining experience, prone to inducing feelings of helplessness. Exercise is a way to fill yourself back up in the face of a difficult situation—for you just as much as for the loved one you are caring for. That's why I often get up extra early, when I know Michael will still be asleep for a couple hours, to fit in my own workout, solo. Michael and I have a good time doing fitness activities together, but to me a time to focus just on myself this way is a treat. Me-time isn't easy to come by for caregivers, but it is absolutely crucial.

Alison's Rules

Alison Morgan, Michael's tennis instructor, has taught me a lot about working with Michael, even though none of her many official certifications and credentials are specific to Alzheimer's disease. Like any good teacher, she is a close observer of her student, and adjusts her approach according to what she sees. Also, she is endlessly upbeat and patient. In addition, Alison is a nationally ranked paddle tennis player. And, not for nothing, she is the granddaughter of a person who had Alzheimer's.

Here are some guidelines I picked up from Alison, aimed at making exercise more accessible and more effective for people with Alzheimer's. And more fun!

- *Notice what is too complicated, and simplify. For instance, drills with more than one ball on the court at a time get confusing, so keep just one ball in motion at a time.*

- *Playing a game is not only a way to make exercise more fun; it also usually involves using your whole body, not just isolated sets of muscles and movements.*
- *Build up complexity gradually over the course of each individual workout, as well as over time. We begin cardio tennis class with arm swings and foot work before we even get out a ball.*
- *Give directions face to face (don't yell out to the group). Even more importantly, demonstrate the desired movement, oriented so that the student can mimic it even if he or she doesn't process what you are saying.*
- *Work on the fly. Flex. Adapt. Adjust. Set the person up for success. Course-correct when you've miscalculated. You might need different strategies on different days.*
- *It doesn't have to be perfect. We're not trying to win any tennis tournaments here; we're just trying to keep our bodies active and healthy, and have fun. If you are moving and having fun, you're doing it correctly!*

How Much Exercise?

Expert advice varies, but the Rush University Medical Center here in Chicago recommends at least 30 minutes of moderate activity daily as best for the brain. We learned two even simpler measures of "enough" from Jason Foster, our trainer: Am I moving my body? Am I breaking a sweat?

For Michael and me, our choice is to exercise more than 30 minutes at a time—and while we are specifically "working out" once a day, we are almost always doing at least two active things in a day. For us, that is working. But that won't be for everybody, so, as with everything else, you have to figure what is right for you and your body and your schedule. More strategies for success:

- Build up gradually. Too much too fast could lead to injury. Perhaps even more importantly, it can lead to discouragement or frustration—and cause you to quit exercising. There's no one right way to build up. All you need is a little common sense. The Rush website suggests exercising for just 10 minutes, but doing that three times a day. As you get stronger, you can exercise for longer each time—with or without cutting down on the total number of times per day.
- Check with the professionals. As with starting anything new in regards to your health, it makes good sense to check with your doctor first to get the thumbs up and review any restrictions that might be necessary. If you do have particular physical limitations, you might want to consult a physical therapist or specialized personal trainer for help designing an exercise approach that is right for you, appropriate, challenging, and safe.
- Create a regular schedule for exercise—what you are doing, where, and when. Make exercise a part of your everyday life. Setting a predictable routine is helpful in general to a person with Alzheimer's, and to keeping any exerciser on track. I've found daily exercise is a great way to lend structure to the whole day for Michael and me. We usually kick-start our day with an official "workout" in the morning, and then do some other active thing in the afternoon, like take a long walk outside with the dogs or go on a bike ride. If the weather isn't cooperating, we might just walk the mall.

- Cross-train. The most basic form of cross-training is to get some aerobic exercise and some strength training—and, I'd add, some work on flexibility. Choosing from a wide variety of physical activities makes it likely you'll address some of the problem areas for a person with Alzheimer's: balance, hand-eye coordination, strength, and flexibility. You already know Michael and I have a whole menu of activities that keep us moving and having fun. Even at the gym, we mix things up, making use of all kinds of machines, for example, including biking, rowing, treadmill walking, lifting weights, and classes like spin and other cardio workouts. Yoga is great, and we plan to do more of it. Your list will be different, depending on what you like to do, what you have experience with, what you have access to, and what you decide to learn. But the key thing is to get exercise in a variety of ways. That is its own form of brain stimulation (tennis is surely lighting up the brain in a different way from something more repetitive like swimming laps or something more meditative, like walking in nature). And it prevents boredom, and so increases the chances that you'll keep on moving.
- Enhance the experience. Get outdoors. Use music. Involve others, including pets! Choose an activity you enjoy. It's like the difference between scarfing down a salad at your desk for lunch because it's good for you and enjoying a meal of your favorite foods with your favorite people with just the right CD playing in the background and a view of the sun setting. Which one are you more eager to do again and again? Biking outside is at the top of Michael's list—who doesn't feel great in fresh air?—along with playing Frisbee with the dogs.

Dress for Success

I'm a big believer is dressing the part—if you go on the court in some crisp tennis whites, I think it gives a little boost to your game. You look like a tennis player and you feel like a tennis player.

When Michael and I exercise, we are never in torn sweats and ratty tee-shirts. Okay, so it's also because I love style, and I enjoy wearing a cute workout outfit. It doesn't have to be some designer—if there was a red carpet leading into the gym, my answer to "Who are you wearing?" would often be "Tar-zhay" (Target). Though I will admit that I adore Lululemon as well.

The right clothes for the occasion can also directly enable a successful workout, like bike shorts with the strategic padding or a headband that will keep your ears warm—and keep you outside longer. The right clothes can ensure safety, like a hoodie with no strings and so nothing to catch on equipment. For Michael and me, clothes can actually be a bonding experience. We have some "his-and-hers" workout gear and that bit of matching is a symbolic way of showing we're working together, that we're on the same team.

Safety First

Safety is one of the reasons to check in with your healthcare provider before beginning any new exercise efforts. But there are several basic things to be mindful of:

- Make sure exercise takes place in a safe environment: plenty of room to move, no hazards, nothing that could get broken. What specifically this means in practice may shift over time.

- Dress appropriately. Layers allow you to remove clothing as your body heats up—and ensure that you won't get too cold in the meantime. You also want to make sure you're not wearing anything that could trip you up, get caught in a machine, or restrict movement.
- Invest in good gym shoes.
- Have water on hand. Make sure all exercisers stay hydrated during and after a workout.
- Start simple and gradually increase number, type, and complexity of exercises.
- Make sure to warm up.
- Always include a cooldown. This is a good time for a drink of water and some chatting.
- Have a plan for adjusting to any limitations.
- Stop if it doesn't feel good. Let your mantra be "No pain. Period."

Jason's Way

Jason's official credentials as a physical trainer also don't cover Alzheimer's, but he has dug in and done his own research about brain conditions and their impact on exercise. Still, as he explains, it wasn't instantly easy for him to work with Michael. It took a little time for them to connect, but that only motivated Jason more. At the beginning, Jason and Michael had a big communication gap, and both tended to end up frustrated. Michael needed to get used to Jason, and with a greater comfort level came better performance. But even more importantly, Jason needed to change his game plan, designing workouts specifically for Michael and figuring out the best ways to teach him. His dedication to being the best teacher to this particular student has really paid off, so I'm going to share some of the strategies I learned from him:

- *Tailor the activity to the person, understanding his or her strengths and weaknesses.*
- *Learning happens by repetition. Maybe a lot of repetition. Repetition is good!*
- *Act more like a workout partner, less like a trainer. Jason moves around the gym with Michael, demonstrating rather than explaining particular moves. Most of the time, the two of them do the exercises together at the same time. I've noticed that other people often watch their workout—it looks fun, like a game!*
- *Keep the person with Alzheimer's in a "safe zone." If Michael starts to get frustrated, he gets defensive, and Jason always takes blame for any misunderstanding on himself. It shifts the vulnerability from Michael to Jason instead, and that lowers the tension and lets Michael move on and make his best effort.*
- *Let go of your own frustration. At first, Jason found he was repeating himself over and over with Michael and getting nowhere, and the more frustrated he got, the more uneasy Michael got. My jovial husband could get downright snippy! This isn't their usual pattern anymore, but with new or challenging exercise it can come up. Jason's go-to solution is to take a "break" to throw around a ball for a few minutes. Michael's still exercising (and practicing that contralateral movement, thank you very much), but having fun, and he can shake off whatever he needs to shake off. So can Jason!*

- *Focus on functional movements. One of the points of exercise is to be able to stay strong in everyday movements. So Jason works with Michael on basic stuff like bending at the knees properly. For this same reason, a lot of what they do targets "contralateral" movement because opposite arm-opposite leg is a foundational pattern of human movement.*
- *Focus on fluid movements. In Alzheimer's, movements often become stiff or rigid; regular practice can counter this effect and keep movement easier for longer.*
- *Don't get too intense with the cardio. One of the main goals here is to get oxygen flowing to the brain, and if too much is demanded by the muscles, you're working at cross-purposes.*
- *Get goofy. Exercise aims to accomplish serious goals, but it doesn't have to be serious business. Michael always goes right along with it when Jason fools around a bit, fake sparring or making something into a silly dance move. Anything to engage a person and keep it fun!*

Find the Right Gym/Teacher/Trainer/Class

One way to know a gym is right for you is if it is convenient. You want one that makes it as easy as humanly possible for you to get there, park, manage your stuff, and so on. The more convenient it is, the fewer obstacles stand in the way of actually using your gym membership.

Exercising can certainly be a do-it-yourself project, but if you are going to join forces with anyone to guide you, you need to choose wisely. Working with the right person will absolutely make all the difference. This also means that if you start a program with someone and it's not a good experience, you should not necessarily give up on that activity.

Look for a good communicator, and a flexible one, who can adjust his or her usual style if necessary. With Michael, for example, a loud voice is a no-go. You need someone who is flexible overall. He or she may need to change up usual methods or existing lesson plans or familiar exercises. You *don't* need someone who already knows all about Alzheimer's, but you do need someone who is empathetic, patient, observant, and willing to learn. And someone who is comfortable around the student; for a lot of individuals, dementia is just too scary or poorly understood, and they aren't going to cope well. You don't need any more complications in your life.

Watch a prospective coach work with other people, if you can, to get a feel for his or her natural style and overall demeanor. You are probably going to need someone who is obviously friendly.

The other half of the equation is the communication *you* need to provide, but the gist is that you need to pave the way with honest communication. Before Michael joined the cardio tennis class, I spoke to the teacher (Alison), of course, but I also reached out to the other people in the class to give them a heads up. I've talked to just about everyone at the gym about Michael, not just Jason, so that people understand what's going on. If Michael forgets his locker combination, someone (male) at the desk will definitely be able to help him with it. If he leaves his phone behind, someone has always scooped it up by the time I call asking after it. I give plenty of credit to Equinox for all the support they've given us (thank you!), but my larger point is that if you don't talk about it, others won't know how to help. So talk!

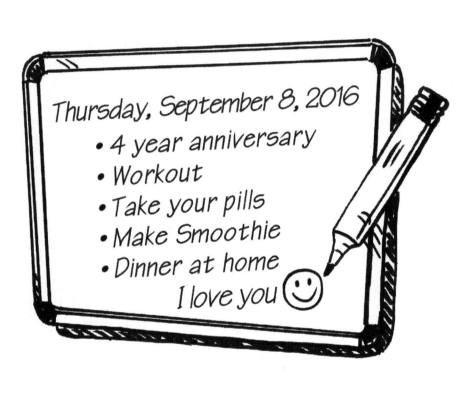

CHAPTER 7

GET ORGANIZED

My brother-in-law called me the day after he returned home from a week at our house in Florida. "I came downstairs this morning and went into the kitchen to check the whiteboard," he told me. Except *his* kitchen doesn't have a whiteboard. He'd gotten so accustomed to seeing it at our house, and now he missed that board.

Michael and I could never be without our whiteboards. There's one in our bathroom and one in our kitchen, and they are absolutely key to keeping us on track. I update them both first thing every morning.

Getting and staying organized becomes more and more challenging for a person with Alzheimer's. Using erasable whiteboards and the other strategies described in this chapter will help keep your days running smoothly, which will, hopefully, reduce your stress. It will help establish and maintain a routine, which is key for a person with Alzheimer's. Further, being organized leads to becoming better oriented, another stress reducer.

These strategies achieve two important goals: they support a person with Alzheimer's *and* provide as much independence as possible. The idea is not to baby our loved ones, but to empower them by creating ways to lessen the effects of limitations that accompany the disease. It's about creating an environment in which they can be successful and feel a sense of personal responsibility and self-confidence.

The less a skill is called upon, the less it is needed and used. This leads to deterioration of the skill. That goes double for awareness and memory. A person who can remind himself what's on tap for the day, or what day of the week it is, or when he'll next see the doctor, benefits from the independence. First, it makes the experience less embarrassing, frustrating, and disempowering. And second, each time an Alzheimer's patient does something independently, it boosts that person's ability to do it again in the future. Without the whiteboards and the related strategies in this chapter, I don't think Michael would still be as engaged as he is four years into this disease.

The strategies in this chapter have definitely saved our day many, many times, and I'm sharing them because I hope they'll be equally powerful for you. Of course, everyone's situation is different, so it only makes sense for you to pick and choose what's right for you. Try things out; keep the ones that work for you and toss what's not helpful. I'm sure you'll come up with additional strategies on your own, which will help you stay innovative. With this disease, things can change from one day to the next, and then change back again. Something that works today might not do the trick tomorrow. This may be due to a temporary glitch or because symptoms have simply progressed. In either case, you'll need to figure out another way to plug the dam. The main points we're sharing have worked fairly well, but we're constantly tweaking the system.

So, Those Whiteboards ...

I swear other organizational tips are coming, but whiteboards rule our world enough that I have to start with those. Their original purpose was to convey practical information, but they also literally show how we take things one day at a time. With this disease, that's an absolute necessity.

I started with a whiteboard prominently displayed in our kitchen. (These boards and the erasable markers used with them are inexpensive, and you can find them at places like Staples, Target, and Walmart.) We are in the kitchen first thing every morning, so getting a look at the whiteboard there is a sure thing. Every morning, with an erasable marker, I write the day and date, including the day of the week and the year. I also give a little note with some kind of reminder of the season, like "beautiful fall day" or "brrrr!" Michael can no longer follow the calendar or time consistently, and that's a totally typical skill to fail early on in this process. But with the whiteboard always displaying the date—and always available for a quick and unobtrusive check—Michael doesn't have stress about what day it is or beat himself up because he doesn't remember.

Under the day and date, I write little reminders like "Take pills" or "Make smoothie" (which sometimes includes some of his medicine).

An outline of the day follows: where we're going, who's coming over, where we're eating, what's on tap for entertainment. It might look something like:

- Workout at club
- 10 a.m. Lee coming over—golf
- Mah-jongg for Cheryl
- Dinner at home
- Monday Night Football (Yay!)

I always include some cute little notes like that "Yay!" Michael is sometimes frustrated when he realizes he's forgotten something, and

I find this approach usually heads that off, because the information is on hand and presented in a light way.

I always include my schedule on the whiteboard as well as Michael's. That's partly so he knows when we're going to be together and when we'll be doing separate activities, not unlike other couples. But there's another reason I do this: the whiteboard is "ours" and not something we do just for Michael. We both make use of this tool so that Michael doesn't feel he's different from everyone else.

The final piece of the whiteboard process is to sign off with "I love you" and a smiley face. I do this every day.

Checking the whiteboard is, at this point, instinctive for Michael. Our eyes automatically go there when we walk through the door, just as my brother-in-law's did after he had been at our house in Florida. Michael looks there first thing every morning, and checks it throughout the day to know what to expect or to see if there's something that needs to be done. He does not have to waste time or energy worrying about what's coming up or when or whether he's doing the right thing or leaving anything out. Like all our strategies, we use the whiteboard to make it as easy as possible for Michael to manage—and to manage as much as he can.

We rely on the whiteboard so much that I bring one along when we travel. That way we can recreate that same focal point in a hotel room, at his sister's house, or wherever we are.

Maintaining the whiteboard isn't just my project; Michael has a key role too. When an agenda item is completed, he erases it from the board, a responsibility he relishes. After he takes his medicine, he immediately walks over and erases that particular item. When he comes home from an outing with Lee, he similarly updates the whiteboard. This, too, is a deeply ingrained habit and an important way for him to maintain control over his schedule.

We rely on a second whiteboard in our bathroom. This one also displays the day/month/year and includes reminders for daily grooming, which I'll say more about in Chapter 12: Looking and Feeling Good.

Set a Regular Schedule

Keeping a regular schedule is essential, and routine is a must. When Michael is off his regular routine, he is just not as happy and his overall responses may be off, or slower. He's not the only one. For anyone, too much unstructured time can cause a certain kind of anxiety. Having predictable structure can reduce stress and boost mood.

However, not just any schedule will do. You want to make sure it's a thoughtful one and a good fit. Consider this person's affinity for structure. People with Alzheimer's differ in their responses to what's happening around them. We have to ask ourselves questions like: What kind of structure are they used to? What times of day are they at their best? When is energy usually low? How do they enjoy spending their time? What needs to be reinforced? Whenever possible, it's also helpful to include a person with Alzheimer's in the planning of the schedule. For example, every 90 days, Michael has a medical appointment as part of the clinical trials he is in. Neither of us controls the timing of that. But when it's time to set up the next appointment, I ask him: "Would you rather go in the morning or the afternoon?"

You want to create an environment in which your loved one feels secure, with lots of opportunities to be successful. Include necessary (and meaningful) assignments, like household chores and personal care, as well as things that are just for fun. Schedule creative outlets, intellectually stimulating activities, and social time. Don't forget physical activity too. If appropriate, include time for religious or spiritual things, like a church service or meditation practice.

Leave plenty of time for each event, so there's no rushing about creating extra pressure. For example, include time for rest or downtime. Schedule activities at regular times, like waking up at 7 or 8 a.m., going to sleep at 10 or 11 p.m., and walking the dogs at 9 a.m. and 4 p.m. Routine is essentially made up of lots of little habits, like the way Michael watches "Squawk Box" every morning to track the stock market. This is routine because he's done this for years and always at the same time every day.

In addition to those routines, we include at least one main activity every day: art on Wednesday, golf on Thursday, music on Friday, and so on. Keeping busy—but not hectic—is what I aim for. Every night I make a plan for what the next day holds. Each morning, I announce the plan for the day (and put it on the whiteboard).

At the same time, you need to remain flexible and adapt to whatever a given day might bring. (Yes, I'm telling you to *plan* for spontaneity.) You'll always be monitoring what's working—and not—and adjusting accordingly.

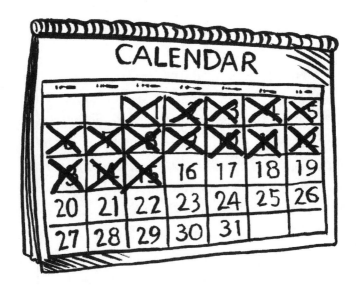

Calendar

It's common for someone with Alzheimer's to confuse what day, week, or year it is. That's one of the reasons we use a large monthly calendar and why, each morning, I cross off the previous day.

We keep this calendar in a prominent spot close to the whiteboard so we can easily check against the date at the top of the whiteboard. When Michael catches me forgetting to cross off a day, he gets a kick out of correcting it.

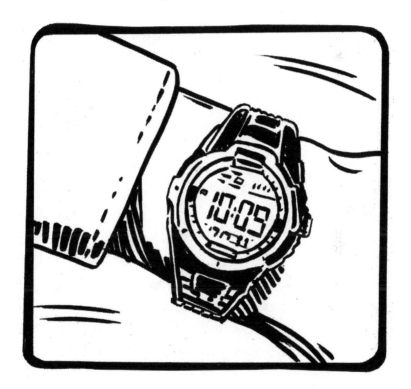

Time

Keeping track of time is another skill that commonly slips early on with Alzheimer's. It took me a little while to realize that Michael's initial difficulties with time were related not just to how his brain was working, but also to the timepieces he used. So we said goodbye to fancy watches with classic analog faces and hello awesome *digital* watches. Telling time is much more straightforward that way. Digital clocks at home have been helpful for the same reason.

Now, however, reading even digital numbers is beyond Michael's ability, but the watch is still important. For one, he is one of those guys who always wore a watch as a style statement. For now, the expensive antique ones are put away so that we don't risk losing them. But something cool-looking on his wrist is still part of Michael's "Michael-ness." Retaining as many habits and lifestyle choices as possible provides a feeling of security.

Laminated Card

One of my first projects on this journey was to make and laminate a small card with lists of important numbers for Michael to keep with him at all times. Imagine a luggage tag. This allowed him to complete ordinary daily transactions independently for much longer than he could have if he had to keep all those numbers in his head. Alzheimer's also impacts one's ability to use numbers. Finding a way to empower Michael in this area for as long as possible was a priority.

I simply printed out copies of the list in an appropriate size and had them laminated at Staples. (Another option is to invest in your own laminating machine; they aren't expensive.)

I put the card on his key chain, and in his wallet (for as long as he still carried a wallet and keys). Actually, I put cards on *all* of the key chains and in *all* of the wallets. I have extras of *everything*. That way, when something goes missing, I can replace it while we look for the stray. This means one fewer layer of stress.

For anyone still driving, keeping a copy of this card in the car is also important. With cards at every turn, Michael can quickly reference our home phone number, my cell, his PIN, home address, date of birth, last four digits of his social security number, contact numbers, and the number you may not realize you are asked for most often: zip code.

Paperwork

If you don't know this already, you surely will find out: you will need to manage a tremendous amount of paperwork for your loved one. I recommend that you seek out professional help, but that's the subject of Chapter 16: Be Proactive: Legal, Financial, and Long-Term Care Planning.

Here I want to share what you can do at home to keep this part of your life as painless as possible:

- Proactively give copies of the relevant medical, legal, and financial reports and records to professionals you work with on a regular basis. If possible, get copies to a family member outside your household too.
- I am big on making extra copies of everything and keeping them in an easily accessible file so that when you need to send something (again) to the insurance company, or to another doctor's office, or when you need to double check something yourself, you can just grab and go. I keep extra hard copies so I can mail one off as necessary without a separate trip to Staples to get a photocopy. I also scan everything into my computer files, so it's easy to email too.
- Keep a list of key contacts—doctors, insurance company, caregivers, instructors—easily accessible. (We have it on the refrigerator.) This is another good laminating project. But do be sure to keep updating your master list.
- Keep an "active" folder with everything you need to bring to doctor's appointments, including a copy of your insurance card, contact info you might need to pass along, reports or instructions from other doctors, any power of attorney or healthcare POA forms, and so on.
- Make (and stick to) a system for documenting your passwords. I use the theoretically risky but more feasible strategy of using the same password for just about everything. Still, I write them all down, especially because it seems you are required to change them frequently.
- Passwords, part II: Make sure that everyone who should have passwords has the ones they need and that you update that group each time you change a password. Or update your

own list and send a new copy to whomever needs it. If you get sick or must travel for an emergency, you will want the person covering for you to have easy access to everything he or she needs.

Charging Electronics

If you haven't already done so, set up a spot devoted to charging phones and other electronics. At a certain time every day, or a certain point in your routine, let it be charging time. When we come home for the day, the first thing we do is plug in. Some people do it as part of getting ready for bed, or at some other convenient time. Just pick what works in your schedule so you'll be able to count on it getting done. (Remember, you can't use the app Find My iPhone if the phone's battery is not charged up…and you're going to need to find your iPhone or, of course, your favorite mobile device—trust me.)

Medication

Creating a system for tracking medications is a total necessity. Often, a pill organizer is all it takes. I have an impressive one that lets me set up three weeks' worth at one time. Make refills a regular part of your routine—every other Monday, say. This gives you plenty of time to note when medications are running low, and to refill them. I do 90-day refills whenever possible and try to keep all medications on a similar schedule so that the entire process can be completed at one time.

Be sure you create a routine for actually *taking* the medicines as well. Michael's medications are mostly taken with food, and our routine is for me to put the right ones out on Michael's placemat at the table so that he can take them as soon as he sits down to eat. It's important not to rely strictly on memory. You will have a lot to keep track of, and it helps to create a habit.

Packing to Go

I've taken over the job of assembling whatever Michael needs when he goes out. I pack his gym bag, for example, with the appropriate change of clothes, hairbrush, deodorant, earbuds, and so on. But then we always go through it together, so he will be confident he has all he needs. It is also a chance for him to run through the process, giving him a bit of ownership.

Part two is taking that packed bag downstairs and placing it in a certain spot near the door. Again, we've established a ritual that has become second nature for both me and Michael. Michael always checks the spot to see if there's anything he should take with him when he heads out.

Color-Coded Closet

Getting dressed is another common challenge. A serious closet makeover has helped Michael immensely. Now, all his clothes are grouped according to type of item—not just shirts one place and pants another, but workout shorts on one shelf, with casual shorts somewhere else, and workout pants in yet another section. T-shirts over here, polos over there, with the appropriate labels on the shelves. If you can, invest in a label maker; it will make so many of these strategies easier to accomplish.

Everything is organized by color too. Overall selection is limited; what he picks will almost always match (or at least not clash). I store out-of-season clothes somewhere else. Also, I pared down the size and variety of his wardrobe. This is why Michael has several white shirts, for example. Before the disease, he had one favorite white shirt. Now, he can wear his favorite color practically every day if he wants. This may seem insignificant, but it makes life a little easier.

Every week when the laundry is done, we work together to put everything back in the designated spot. Each day I clear out dirty clothes, because otherwise they are likely to just end up back in the closet and be reworn the next day. (This is another very common habit for people with Alzheimer's.)

Lost and Found

Part of your new normal will be devoted to finding lost stuff. My advice is to cut down on the hunting-for-stuff part of your life by putting some preventative measures in place. Just as important: try not to become upset when something does get lost; it's just stuff.

The top priority is to designate a specific place to put down small items you use every day. You might already do this to keep track of your own stuff, but it's going to be especially important to make it an explicit system for a person with Alzheimer's. When I take off my watch, for example, I make sure to put it down on my bureau. If I leave it anywhere else and forget to make a mental note of it, I end up wasting time retracing my steps looking all over for it. Fortunately, watch-on-bureau is a pretty deeply ingrained habit for me at this point, so *most* of the time when I want my watch, it is exactly where I first look for it. (I also know my favorite hiding spots, so if something is not where it is *supposed* to be, I know where to check for it. Reading glasses tend to be waiting where I left them on the coffee table, for example, if they haven't made it back to the bureau.)

For all the things we refer to as "Michael's stuff," I have small labeled pottery dishes on the bathroom counter—"watch," "ring," "dog tag"—to designate where objects go. I can't say it *always* works, but it's a good first line of defense, and when he's looking for one of these items, we have a good idea of where to look first. We also rely on Michael's long-established habits, like keeping his wallet and money clip in the top drawer. The difference now is that I need to know Michael's exact habits. Sometimes he follows the habit—he removes his wallet from his pocket and puts it in the drawer as usual. But then he either forgets that he's taken it out of his pocket or that he has a system for doing so. So now that I've tuned in to his habits and routines, I know where to begin the search.

We also store belongings in specific places in the car: sunglasses in the little cavity over the radio, loose change in the cup holder, and so on. (We make a little game for ourselves with the change we collect: when the stash gets big enough, we take it to the mall for a fun, low-stakes shopping spree.)

Follow the Leader
I literally tag along after Michael and watch where he puts things around the house, especially when we come home from an outing and when he's getting ready for bed—and any time he's taking things out of his pockets. I watch where he puts stuff and if it's anywhere other than the usual, I make a mental note of it. I don't move

anything, but this way if he doesn't remember I can help retrace his steps with him.

So that Michael doesn't become confused, I don't move misplaced items to the spot where they belong. He may return to the spot where he left something and reclaim it. That's okay. Also, when something is temporarily missing, Michael is likely to say that someone has taken it—a common response. I simply show him where he's put the item. Sometimes this jogs his memory enough so that he understands no one else has taken his belonging. Occasionally, when this happens—when he thinks something has been stolen, which can be upsetting—I reassure him that the object is not gone and that we'll find it together. "Let's check our places" is our shorthand for this. Then I turn our search into a game—a treasure hunt—which usually defuses his frustration.

Watching where Michael puts stuff also helps me when it comes time to find a "missing" item. Paying attention this way also allows me to discover when he's developed a new habit or routine. If I notice enough times that he's begun to place his watch on the kitchen counter, then I know that's where to find it (versus the "watch" dish in our bathroom). I also have to pay attention to where Michael stashes items in the car.

Extra! Extra!

Here's one of the strategies that has significantly reduced frustration for both of us: we get extra copies of important items Michael uses on a daily basis—extra sets of keys, wallets, glasses, money clips, even driver's licenses (now that Michael's not driving, he has a state ID instead)—anything, really, that could be lost. Keep several of each on hand and easily available in your home. You'll know right where to go for the replacement instantly and avoid unnecessary stress.

It's important to help the person with Alzheimer's feel like this is no big deal. Having extras on hand helps. I also let him know he's not the only one who misplaces things. I have extra reading glasses in every room, in my purse, and in my car.

Something's Missing

No matter what plans you make, you're not going to keep tabs on everything. So you need some strategies for finding what has been lost.

Remember that supply of extra copies I have? This is why I keep it readily accessible—some upstairs, some downstairs—so I can grab a replacement if we can't find what's missing. This, too, keeps anxiety to a minimum.

Missing items is one of the reasons it is so important to talk to literally everyone in your life about the fact that you're dealing with Alzheimer's. Sharing this particular aspect of the disease makes it easier when you're on the hunt for something left behind.

And let me just add: thank goodness for Find My iPhone. We probably use this app even more than we actually talk on the phone. One of my top priorities is keeping the phone charged up, and turned on, so we can access this tool.

Keep Your Cool

The frequency with which items go missing is obviously going to be frustrating for everyone. But your job as caregiver is to try to keep your frustration under wraps. Frustration is contagious, so if you're displaying yours, your loved one is likely to pick up on that and feel it as well. Acting out your frustration won't do anything to help the situation. I'm not suggesting that you deny your feelings. You are going to need a way to process and/or vent your emotions—more on this in Chapter 10: Care for the Caregiver—but doing so in the heat of the moment isn't helpful.

The second part of your job in this situation is to reassure your loved one that whatever is lost is not *gone*, and that you will find it together (or replace it). Sometimes we make searching for items a bit of a game, and I give "hot" or "cold" clues. Calling on your best understanding of what your loved one is going through will help you empathize and clue you in to where those lost items are hiding.

Finally, if something has gone missing, here's what you do: *Let. It. Go.* I know: easier said than done. We've lost iPhones, car keys, photos, passports, mail, and checks. But remember, it's still just stuff.

As always, we're trying to maintain a system that provides all the support needed to minimize frustration, and at the same time allows Michael to handle as much as possible on his own.

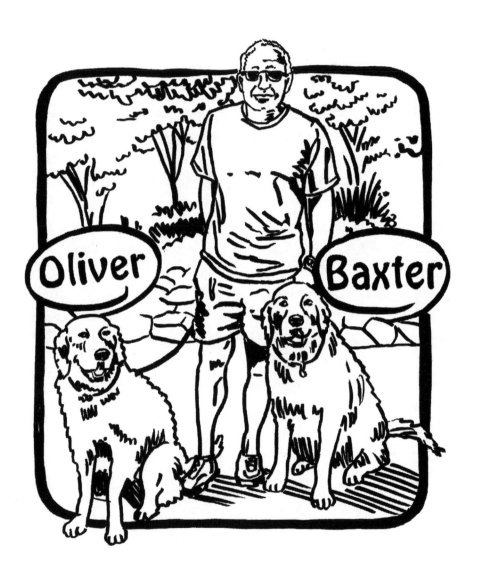

CHAPTER 8

A DOG'S UNCONDITIONAL LOVE

I love this quote by author M.K. Clinton (*The Returns*): "The world would be a nice place if everyone had the ability to love as unconditionally as a dog." Here's how you know it's *true* love: picture Michael all bundled up heading out into a Chicago winter day, just so Oliver can play in the snow. Or imagine me dealing with all the cleaning products required to housebreak puppy Oliver. Or maybe the most telling detail is the way Oliver quivers all over when he sees Michael after they've been apart for a little while; this dog bounds over to him as soon as he gets half a chance. These two share a really wonderful bond.

It's that emotional bond that puts getting Oliver—and later, his younger brother, Baxter—at the top of the list of what's really worked for Michael. Dogs offer unconditional love, and Oliver and Baxter are definitely not afraid to show it. Oliver, particularly, offers comfort and a calming influence just by his presence, which is influenced by his Emotional Support Animal Training. (Baxter is a bit more of a wild one, so although he has many wonderful qualities, being a *calming* influence is not really one of them.)

The physical contact, we've discovered, is as important and effective as the emotional connection that comes with having dogs in the family. Lack of touch is devastating to anyone, particularly someone suffering with Alzheimer's. But Michael and Oliver share physical affection, and that kind of connection is priceless. Oliver is almost always touching Michael when they are together. People who see them together often notice the way Oliver leans into Michael or gets calmly between Michael and any person who approaches him.

The dogs create a lot of opportunities for socializing too. Working with the dog trainer is social; being out and about with a friendly dog facilitates social interaction with the people you come across, and the dogs themselves are social. So any time you hang out with them you are socializing. Plus, Oliver and Baxter keep Michael company, which shields him from some of the loneliness people with Alzheimer's are at risk for.

Taking care of the dogs is a responsibility—at a time when so many responsibilities are being removed—and a meaningful way to spend time. Plus, it's *fun* being with Oliver. Just being around him makes Michael smile and laugh. The dogs bring out a playful side of Michael, which is one of the reasons *I* enjoy them. Having dogs to care for also encourages him to get fresh air and exercise; even people who don't get up off the couch for their own well-being will do it for their dogs. Michael is very active anyway, with or without the dogs, but they are a great outlet when he really *needs* to be active and to let off steam. For a long time, when he would start pacing the house, stirred up about who knows what, the best solution was to send him on a long walk with Oliver and Baxter.

Hanging with an emotional support dog like Oliver reduces stress and improves mood, decreasing anxiety and depression. Science can prove it: measures include lowered blood pressure and lowered heart rates.

Actually, you can get most of the above benefits from any pet, no matter what the animal or training. For us, though, the "emotional support" specialization has been really important. It's worth noting that any animal can be an emotional support animal—emotional support iguana, anyone?—though for us, a dog was the way to go. In a different living situation, maybe a cat would make more sense, or a smaller dog. (If an animal is a no-go for you for whatever reason, you can even tap into a lot of the benefits by caring for *plants*. You may not get cuddles, but there's responsibility, a meaningful way to keep busy, fresh air and exercise, and possibility for social interaction around the subject.) As with so much else, you have to find what best fits your circumstances.

Service and Therapy Animals

I know a lot of people use these terms interchangeably with "emotional support animal," but there are important technical differences between all of them. Here are the basic jobs of each:

- Service dogs are trained to perform specific tasks for their owners, such as "seeing-eye" dogs that guide vision-impaired people, or diabetes service dogs that provide alerts for low blood sugar.
- Therapy dogs receive specific training to go with their owners to visit and work with people in hospitals, schools, nursing homes, disaster areas, and the like.

- Emotional support dogs provide…emotional support. Just by being around, they are calming and comforting.

Carol Ross, Certified Dog Trainer, Canine Dimensions

I started working with Oliver when he was about eight weeks old. The window for socializing puppies runs until they are about five months old. My first goal was to get Oliver up to American Kennel Club "Good Canine Citizen" standards. I wanted him to have good manners, be polite, and act appropriately wherever he went, no matter whom he was with. He had a little more training specific to being an Emotional Support Animal, so he'd stay close to Michael, literally touching him much of the time, place his head on Michael's lap to help keep Michael calm as needed, and do things like "hold stay" for two hours so he could go on plane trips.

We were laying the groundwork for all of this starting at two months old. But the key piece when he was so young was introducing him to as many people and situations as possible. While working with me, he was exposed to at least 300 people, 60 friendly dogs, and a wide range of environments, medical equipment, and behaviors. We went to all kinds of dog-friendly events, stores, schools, and parks, anything I could think of. We spent time downtown. We went to the airport.

A lot of this socialization was before he began to work on specific skills with Michael. In the early days, their job together was just to form a strong bond. After that, we started the more formal "obedience" training. Normally, I do that over four or five sessions, about one a month. Like humans, dogs learn best when the process is simple. In this case, keeping it simple meant breaking the process down into smaller pieces, taking our time, and allowing for more practice, and more repetitions of each skill. Consistency is the key.

Through this process, Oliver and Michael learned the commands "come," "sit," "down," "stay," and "drop it." In addition, they mastered "look" (for Oliver to make eye contact with Michael), "touch" (for Oliver to gently touch Michael's hand), "enough" (stop what you are doing!), and "away" (give me a little space). Oliver and Baxter both learned "go to your place" for when someone comes to the door who doesn't really need a high-energy canine greeting committee.

This collection of commands covers most things that come up for most dogs and their people. Many dogs need a little additional training in this or that, specific to their situation and depending on their personalities, behavior, and circumstances. A small dog that lives in an apartment and annoys the neighbors with barking can be taught to stop barking on command, for example.

Some dogs are trained specifically as service dogs for people with Alzheimer's, which is mainly to help with a person who wanders or gets lost. But Oliver's job is different—he's for company, calming, and comfort.

Choose the Right Animal Companion
Your first decision will be what kind of animal will be best for your circumstances. A big dog that is able to keep up with a very active lifestyle or a small dog that's easier to take everywhere in a "purse"? Or, if a person with Alzheimer's has always been a "cat person," then

maybe that's the way to go. Then again, a person's interests evolve in interesting ways as a result of this disease, so someone who never much wanted to deal with pets before may now light up just passing a dog in the park. Some people might seem more content sitting quietly with a fluff ball in their laps or trying to keep up with a high-energy critter. A cat might be a better choice than a dog for living in an apartment and a great option if you want to travel with the animal. Maybe you're going to do better with a hamster. Perhaps pet ownership is not for you, but you can arrange regular visits from a therapy dog. Just watching a fish tank or a bird feeder can be a calming, relaxing experience, even if it doesn't exactly bring the same kind of bonding component you'd get with a dog or cat.

You also want to think about who will be the primary caregiver, how much energy he or she can devote to the job, and their preferences for the type of animal selected. You want the person with Alzheimer's to contribute to the caretaking of the animal, but someone will need to keep tabs on things and step in as necessary.

Oops!

In a weak moment, about a year after we got Oliver, I agreed to take in his full brother (same parents, different litter) too. Baxter turned out to be a bit of a handful. You know how older siblings are the overly responsible ones, and younger siblings tend to be more free-spirited? Apparently that's a thing in English Crème Golden Retrievers as well as people.

I jokingly refer to Baxter as my "oops!" baby, but, really, he's a welcome addition to the family. He's "my" dog, the way Oliver is Michael's, although somehow when it is time for a walk in the middle of a Chicago winter, they are suddenly both mine! If that's not enough to show you how much I love him, consider the fact that he is still with us even after the day he ate every last one of my orchids! While I adore Baxter, sometimes adding a pet is like suddenly having a new child, so do think carefully before bringing in a second pet.

It's good for the dogs to have each other's company too (even though I'm pretty sure Oliver thinks he is a person). The two of them are very close, always get along, and sleep side by side every night.

And here's the benefit of doubling our canine fun that we never planned on: I know there will be a time when Michael can no longer direct Oliver on his own. But I also know from watching what Michael does in other situations that when that day comes, Michael will be able to follow suit with what I do with Baxter. Oliver will always be tied to Michael, come what may, commands or no commands. But the longer Michael can still be "in charge" of Oliver, the better. Having a model he can copy—a lead he can copy—will be a key way for Michael to manage that.

Choose the Right Dog

Once we decided to get a dog, I searched online for information on the dog breeds that are the best match for people with Alzheimer's; mainly I was looking for loving, comforting dogs. The Internet is packed with different discussions on specific breeds, and that's what led me to the Old English Crème golden retriever. They are very gentle dogs that bond readily and strongly with their people. Breeds that are generally smart, good communicators, and eager to please are good choices, and, of course, there's more than just one breed that meets these requirements.

When it comes to individual dogs, you're looking for all those same things, although not every Old English Crème is calm and cooperative like Oliver and Baxter. Above all, you need a solid and *calm* dog, a dog that is, as trainer Carol Ross says, "bomb proof." You want a dog that will roll with whatever comes its way—noise, crowds, a kid pulling its ear—and sit there and "smile," knowing it is safe with its person. Let anxious or skittish dogs be someone else's project; you have enough on your plate as it is and don't want to be providing emotional support *to* the animal. Achieving the right fit for your situation makes all the difference.

Getting the right dog also means finding the appropriate source for your dog. If you are looking for a specific breed, you are likely going to be getting a dog from a breeder. This means you need to make sure you work with a responsible breeder, one who breeds for health and temperament, and not just looks. Veterinarians and trainers may be a good source of referrals. You're going to need a vet eventually, and probably want a trainer too, so why not start your search for a dog by finding people to help you care for the one you ultimately bring home? Then let them help guide your choice.

Gimme Shelter

Mixed breeds can make great emotional support animals too, and you can find the perfect support animal at a shelter. Adopting an animal is generally a more budget-friendly way to go. Plus, you get the satisfaction of giving a home to a dog (or cat) that really needs one.

The trick, as always, is to find the right combination of temperament and traits for the job you want the animal to do.

Carol Ross advises talking with the staff at a shelter to let them know you're looking for an emotional support animal. They know the animals well and can help guide your selection, but not if they don't understand your specific goals. Or ask a knowledgeable trainer to accompany you and help you select a dog. (That is also a good option if you're going to a breeder.)

Puppies!

I'm not going to lie: puppies are a lot of work. And you really don't need an additional challenge in your life right now. That said, to get the closest bond and the optimal socialization and training, starting early is a great benefit. You may have to think creatively here. Depending on your circumstances, maybe puppy-raising actually is a great project for you to take on with your loved one. But if not, maybe there's a close friend or family member who could "foster" the puppy. You're looking for a situation that will allow plenty of bonding time between the puppy and the person with Alzheimer's. (There are nonprofit groups that train and provide dogs, but wait time is long, costs are high, and they may be doing more training than what is strictly necessary for an emotional support animal.)

Do I Really Need a Trainer?

We chose to work with Carol to achieve particular behaviors from Oliver. Our relationship with Carol has turned into a longer lasting one than what occurs during most training periods. First, it's good for Michael to keep practicing, and, second, Michael and Oliver need some new skills over time as the situation shifts. But it doesn't have to be that big of an investment in time or money to have a trainer guide you in getting your dog ready to earn the 10-point AKC "Canine Good Citizen" designation.

You might be able to do the training as part of a class, but for someone with Alzheimer's it would probably have to be a very small class. If you think the social aspects would outweigh the potential distractions of increased noise and activity in the room, a group situation may be a good (and cheaper!) option.

Either way, investing in some help at the outset of your relationship with your dog can make a significant difference in the long run. Down the road, you may need backup assistance to care for your pets. Don't hesitate to ask for help from friends, family, and neighbors. Also, check your vet and/or local pet supply stores for doggie daycares in your area.

Dogs Are Kind of Zen

Finally, dogs are nonjudgmental. They live in the moment. These are great gifts to someone living with Alzheimer's. A little unconditional calm and comfort is probably a great thing for the caregivers who get to spend time around them too.

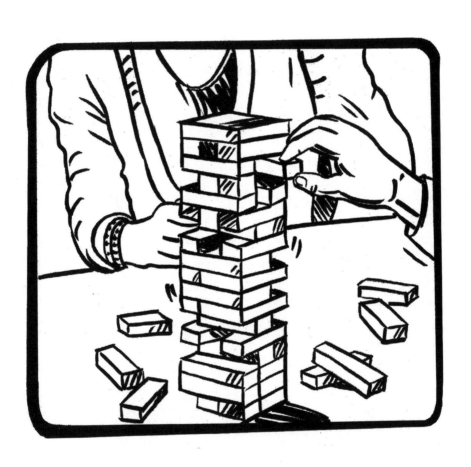

CHAPTER 9

BRAIN WORK

As you may know, crossword puzzles—and other word games—can help keep your brain active, especially as you age. Anything and everything that stimulates the brain helps, including exercising, socializing, and creative pursuits. All kinds of activities light up various areas of the brain, so mixing and matching as many mentally stimulating activities as possible is the way to go.

In our first meeting with Dr. Yucus, he did, in fact, recommend doing puzzles and, in general, anything that would stimulate brain health. Based on his advice, Michael and I include all kinds of activities in our daily lives. Many of the activities discussed in this chapter serve multiple purposes, from fostering social interaction to promoting physical activity—both of which stimulate the brain.

Memory Montage
One evening, as Michael and I watched the movie *50 First Dates* with Drew Barrymore and Adam Sandler, I was inspired to make a "memory montage" for Michael. In this movie, Drew Barrymore has suffered a brain injury and loses all her short-term memory. Every day needed to be a reminder of how wonderful her life once was. Every

date with Adam Sandler is like their first. It's an inspiring movie, one I strongly suggest.

Creating the montage is one of the best decisions I've ever made in our new normal life. Like the videos we've all seen at weddings and bar/bat mitzvahs, a memory montage is a series of photos of significant people, places, and times in Michael's life, and the images are set to music he knows and loves. While Chicago songs—like "Beginnings" by the band Chicago—play, the montage features video and photos from our wedding. I also included pictures of Michael when he was young, vacations, family and friends, and milestones like birthday parties, graduations, and holidays. Michael especially likes the photographs that trace his family history. Seeing where he came from brings him much joy. He also loves the testimonials from his cousins recorded for Michael's fifty-eighth birthday party.

Michael watches the montage several times a week, singing along as he watches the story about his life—including our time together—unfold, perfectly synced with meaningful lyrics. The music is key to getting and keeping him engaged as he reviews the memories. Our montage evolves as our life changes and as we add more milestones, like our trip to Italy.

Michael frequently watches the video, which, I believe, preserves special, positive memories. Playing the video—and watching together—is an important part of our routine. We chat about the video before, during, and after it runs, and often the memories featured elicit additional remembrances.

We also have lots of photos around the house, and other mementos like the shells we collected on the beach at our wedding celebration. Whenever possible, use props to facilitate reminiscing. Photo albums and old songs are typical examples, but any meaningful object can help. Sensory stimulation occasionally stirs memories too, like the smell of an ocean breeze or the taste of a favorite food from childhood. Anything—a song, a photograph, a spoken memory—can be used as a springboard to reminisce. Enjoying good memories also can build up strength for getting through some of the tough times.

Have Fun

Having fun may be the best way to engage a person with Alzheimer's. Explore hobbies and activities he or she loves and commit to doing something fun every day.

Is gardening fun for you? Do that. Crosswords? Ping-pong? Singing in a choir? Do those things. For Michael and me, one of the most reliable ways to put a shot of enjoyment into our day is to play games. We're not talking chess, though we do play backgammon with quite an original set of rules. We also love card games, Jenga, Twister, Pictionary, and more. Games serve as an instant mood-changer around here. Games also provide rich social opportunities. The best games are the ones we can play with other people. Often, these games are more popular than dinner parties. For instance, the basic Toys "R" Us bingo set has become an excellent investment in fun.

Here's a piece of advice you won't find in most books about Alzheimer's: try "drunk Jenga"! All you need is a bottle of wine or a couple martinis, a group of people, and that tower of wooden blocks. Getting drunk is not actually required, but a glass of wine or a dirty martini does make the game more…challenging. And it is a great equalizer! (And if any of that strikes you as too risqué, definitely do *not* ask me about how Michael and I sometimes use Twister to help plan activities for later in the evening …).

Laugh Often

Michael and I love to laugh, something I believe should be part of every day. Sure, laughing is probably not the first thing that pops to mind when I say "living with Alzheimer's." Truthfully, however, if I weren't laughing, I'd probably be crying. Without humor, this disease has too much sadness. You have to find laughter wherever you can get it. And if you can't find it, create some laughter on your own. I think humor and laughing provide multiple ways to stimulate the brain, from the work involved in "getting" a joke to the experience of shifting a mood.

Michael and I laugh together all the time. Sometimes, it's just at something we see out in the world that strikes us as funny. Other times, I admit, it's an Alzheimer's-induced situation that makes us laugh. If you can't laugh about finding a set of keys in the freezer, what can you laugh about? Sometimes we engage in an activity already proven to elicit laughter, like playing Pictionary.

Occasionally, we seek laughs delivered by comedians (a live show or something on TV), funny movies, and sitcoms. Make sure you select suitable material, because jokes that go over a person's head aren't going to provoke laughter. I observe Michael watching television programs and judge by his reactions how well he's following the material. For comedies, I want to see if he's laughing at appropriate times. If that's not the case, we choose another show. Our longtime favorite is *Big Bang Theory* because the jokes are natural to the scenes and nobody is talking too fast. For example, the silly behavior of the characters reminds us of one of our friends—every time Sheldon does something silly, we burst out laughing. That's how I know Michael is still connected. *Friends* is another favorite around here for similar reasons.

Regardless of how or why it starts, laughter is an uplifting, bonding, and social experience, all of which benefits the brain.

If I get sad, I always have to think of something that will make me laugh. —Michael

---

Chores

Doing chores serves a similar purpose when it comes to stimulating the brain. Chores can be anchor points for maintaining structure and routine—feeding the dog each morning or taking the trash out to the curb every Tuesday. Chores are meaningful work and provide everyone an opportunity to contribute to running the household. Chores are familiar, everyday activities, and keeping up as many of those as possible is beneficial. Chores completed independently provide a sense of responsibility. Approaching chores as a team offers a great form of socialization. Some chores can even be a form of exercise, depending on how you do them.

Michael has a roster of chores, all of which give him a sense of pride. He takes out the trash each week, collects the mail and the newspaper every day, and cleans out the fireplace as needed. In the mornings, while I set the table for breakfast, he takes out our coffee mugs. After dinner, he clears the table while I put dishes in the dishwasher.

Established routines like chores provide some continuity and "normalcy." If you can maintain the status quo, that will help your loved one. Similarly, if necessary, you can adapt the chores to accommodate any changes in behavior or one's physical limitations. For example, you might need to simplify a chore so that it's more manageable. "Doing the laundry" might simply mean folding the laundry if sorting the colors and choosing the right temperature becomes impractical. At our house, laundry isn't an issue, mostly because I am one of those rare birds who really loves to do laundry. It's my thing, not Michael's, which brings me to my last tip in this category: there's no need to start a person on *new* chores just for the sake of doing chores. Michael is not going to suddenly start making the bed for the first time in our life as a couple *now*. Of course, a person may be more into chores, and eager for responsibilities, in which case you can add whatever he or she can and wants to manage.

Reading

Michael reads *The Wall Street Journal* every day, something he's always done. He loves to comment on various articles and shares those that are related to the industry in which we both worked. He studies the stock pages—another longtime habit—and can still tell you which stocks he has and his opinion about them despite the fact that Alzheimer's can make reading harder and harder as the disease progresses. I suspect that Michael can read as much as he can because he's been doing it for so long. Reading is a great way to stimulate the brain, as long as it doesn't get so frustrating that it creates stress. Also, I've discovered that our discussions are as important to his brain health as the articles he has read.

Michael's at the stage now where he uses his finger to track the words across the page so he doesn't lose his place. This is a new behavior, so I know his skill is slipping. Some people read out loud for similar reasons. None of that means that reading is no longer a good activity. It's unlikely that Michael is going to pick up a copy of *War and Peace*, mostly because he's never really been a big Russian literature guy. But he's still interested in sports, so he keeps up by reading a sports magazine and the daily paper.

I do watch him when he reads, and I can tell when he's not paying attention, which means he's not able to follow it. That's okay if he just backtracks or decides to keep going, but if he looks like he's disengaging then I know it's time for a different activity.

I know he is still taking something from whatever he reads, because he talks to me about certain articles. I remind myself that it doesn't matter if he remembers what he reads; as long as he is engaged while he is doing it, the activity is worthwhile. All that input to the brain has to be good. I know many people enjoy audiobooks, which we haven't really explored much, but it will probably be a good substitute when reading becomes too difficult. Or maybe one day, rather than wait for Michael to toss out tidbits from the paper, I'll read articles to him. One way or another, we'll do our best to tweak and modify our activity so that we can continue with it.

Television

Television features prominently in my worst fears about care available for people with Alzheimer's. The thought of Michael just sitting, zoned out, in front of a television that's never off is horrifying to me. But the truth is, watching television *can* be a good way to add a little more brain stimulation into your life. You don't want to be doing nothing but watching, and you don't want to watch passively.

Discuss what you're watching: talk over the news or discuss the characters on a show. Michael loves anything about stocks, sports, or politics, so we are big ESPN and Fox News fans.

Our routine after dinner is typically to watch a movie or, depending on the time of year, sports. (We never watch TV *during* dinner; that would make it too easy to disengage.) With movies, sports themes are usually the most successful for us. I observe Michael while he watches so that I can make sure he's able to follow the story. We often watch the same movies we've seen before, especially the James Bond films. We both derive all the familiar pleasures of an old movie, and, for Michael, this means less stress on memory. Another strategy is to look for movies and shows that don't depend on plot (the less you have to follow, the easier it is to enjoy), like those with travel or nature themes. For us, another key component is our time together. We snuggle up on the couch together, whatever we're watching. So even though our daily routine is too busy to allow just vegging out with the TV on, television *is* part of our winding-down activity.

Getting Out There

Researchers at the Rush University Medical Center (home to one of this country's leading Alzheimer's research centers) have identified a person's "life space" to be inversely related to their risk of developing Alzheimer's disease: more life space, less risk. (The results of this study were published in the *American Journal of Geriatric Psychiatry*.) "Life space" is how the research describes the degree to which people live their lives outside their own homes—how often they get outside, how often they engage in their community, how often they work or volunteer, how much they garden or walk or just run errands or visit the library. The fascinating thing is that it didn't much matter what activity got people out of their beds or rooms or houses. The more often they were simply out and about, the lower their risk of developing the disease.

I know a lot of people with Alzheimer's and their caregivers who remove themselves from social interaction and stay away from public venues, and the reasons are many. Some are simply embarrassed by the disease. I'm angry at the disease. I wish Michael didn't have the disease. But we are not embarrassed by Alzheimer's. I do everything to preserve Michael's dignity, of course, but much of what might be considered "embarrassing" doesn't register that way for him; it's the person *with* him who might feel embarrassed. But why should I feel embarrassed because he forgets a name, or says something not clearly related to someone else's remark, or makes a social faux pas? This is what talking to everyone about Alzheimer's helps me avoid: what people understand, they can accept as business as usual. And then we can all move on. The only "risk" I recognize about having a person with Alzheimer's out in the world is that too much of anything can be overwhelming. That's when it's time to go home. But we don't *stay* home. The risks of not going out are too great. By staying inside, the chance of disengaging can become 100 percent.

I'm glad to know science backs up my instinct to keep Michael involved with all kinds of things that expand his world and stimulate his brain. I hope you will look for ways to get out as much as possible and enjoy the world beyond your front door.

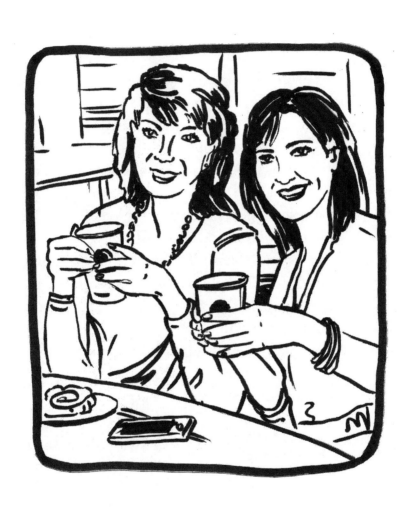

CHAPTER 10

CARE FOR THE CAREGIVER

My close friend and former colleague Andrea once said, "Why are you working? Make your time with Michael count." For a long time, I coordinated Michael's care, managed our life together, worked full time, and ran myself completely ragged trying to do it all. The paperwork alone put me into a semipermanent state of exhaustion.

Then one morning, sitting in a Starbucks, Andrea looked at me and asked, "Cheryl, what are you *doing*? You are so stressed. Why not just retire?" At first, I protested. I loved my job and had never thought of retirement, but I knew she was right. Retiring had literally never crossed my mind; I needed someone else to say, "Don't miss this time."

I realized that I wanted to, literally, *be* there for Michael. Initially, I worked from home, thanks to the FMLA (Family Medical Leave Act), but it was challenging as Michael's condition progressed. I needed to shift my priorities—focus on family and officially retire. I am fortunate that I could afford this decision, but it's still a tricky transition to suddenly retire from the work you love. So much of my identity focused on being a "working mom." And my relationship with Michael extended to our professional lives. After all, we worked together for years. Now, my focus is Michael and my life is in balance. I've learned how to take care of myself, which gives Michael the best of me.

Caregiving is, without question, one of life's biggest challenges, and with so many demands on your time and energy, it's easy to neglect taking good care of yourself. Self-care—figuring out how to stay physically and emotionally strong—turns out to be the best thing you can do for the person you are caring for. But that's not going to happen unless you schedule the time. If you don't plan for it, finding the time will be difficult. So make a commitment to yourself *for* yourself.

Several moving parts need to coalesce for true self-care: physical and mental health, positive mental attitude, stress management, and emotions are all important. It's the same for everyone, of course, but even more urgent for caregivers. The same balance you're striving to ensure for your loved one is what you should be seeking for yourself. It's what you *need* to be seeking if you want to continue to do your most important job. This will look a little bit different for each caregiver, each person being cared for, and each situation and phase. But the general themes are the same: take care of your body, educate yourself, take breaks, find creative and restful outlets, and talk about it.

Take Care of Your Body

You need to look after your own physical health. Eat right. Exercise. Get your sleep. See your doctor regularly. Learn ways to manage your stress. Stay connected to friends and family. Do whatever you have to do to find the time to do these things. Schedule them into your day/week/year. Think creatively; ask a friend to cover for a while so you can attend yoga class or hit the gym. Or exercise at home with a video or an app. Or work out with the person you are caring for—whatever works. Just make sure you do something every day to take care of your body.

Educate Yourself

Stay well informed about Alzheimer's—the disease, best practices, and available resources. If you can't find what you need, dig deeper and ask the professionals for help. Try not to become overwhelmed; spread out your research and give yourself a break. Seek out the right balance between getting the best information you need to navigate successfully and piling on another never-ending responsibility to your already busy life. Try to take it on a need-to-know basis. You need strategies, yes, but you don't need to understand all about the genetics of Alzheimer's or memorize the highlights of the latest study. At some point you may need information about ways to communicate with a person who doesn't talk much, but it's not necessary to obtain the data *right now*. Take it one step at a time.

Take a Break

This is a big guilt-inducer, but it shouldn't be: you're going to need breaks. Nobody can do this job alone 24/7/365. Arrange care, formally or informally, with hired caregivers or friends and family who are game. Mix and match the care to accommodate your situation. Then make regular use of it in large and small ways. Sometimes you may need to get away. I traveled with my daughter for spring break during her senior year of high school while Michael stayed with his sister. Sometimes you may need to "disappear" for a shorter break—time to get to the gym, the hair salon, or whatever makes you feel good. All of this is not only okay; it's mandatory.

Every caregiver needs an outlet. I exercise. That's always been my passion, and I still find time for it every day. I know it's good for me and my health, of course, but for me exercise is also a way to defuse my frustrations and reduce my stress level. I exercise for my *mental* health. The time I spend exercising is also just a plain old break from the rest of my day.

I also play mah-jongg. On Sundays, friends come over so I don't have to leave Michael. On Mondays, I go out to play while Michael spends time with his "buddy" Lee.

These are my favorite ways to leave everything behind for a little while and recharge my batteries. Figure out what helps you decompress and de-stress, whatever hobby or activity it may be, and make a point of including it in your schedule on a regular basis. It can be as simple as coffee with a friend or as complex as a side business—or as simple *and* complex as a great glass of cabernet!

You also can look for ways to unwind *with* the person you are caring for. I found a masseuse who comes to our house so both Michael and I can get a massage. Try walks outdoors, dancing to favorite music—whatever makes you both feel good. We like going for side-by-side pedicures. This kind of joint activity is restorative, too, as long as you make sure it is in addition to, rather than a replacement for, whatever you do just for yourself.

Talk About It

I see a therapist once a week, and it's a safe place where I can talk about my fears. Watching someone you love experience Alzheimer's is frightening and, frankly, sometimes just horrible. If I didn't have someone to talk openly with to process the experience, I worry that I might give up. I think it is important to be honest about your feelings, especially the dark ones, so you don't get trapped by them. You have to own your emotions, or they'll own you. Individual therapy isn't for everyone. Other options include group therapy, support groups, and wise, supportive, and nonjudgmental friends. Sometimes I just need to vent, and I know I can do that with my friends Andrea and Anne. They're always willing to listen.

Dr. Linda Randall

The caregiver for a partner with Alzheimer's disease experiences an ongoing sense of loss; the grieving process may be conscious or buried deep within. Feelings of anger, fear, guilt, sadness, etc. complicate the caregiver's task of needing to manage a complex daily existence for both the caregiver and the partner with diminished functioning. The caregiver is most often responsible for the link to a network of family and friends, guiding them as they transform their relationships with the Alzheimer's patient. The caregiver's emotional and physical energy can become depleted rather rapidly, so it's important that the soul find ways to regenerate inner strength.

Caregivers must find ways to take care of themselves. This life-altering situation begs the caregiver to stay as healthy and balanced as possible. Staying active in one's own life is very important. Continuing as many normal activities as one is able to do, while seeking the companionship of caring, empathic, supportive friends and family, is the broad outline of "what to do."

One of the best ways for caregivers to take care of themselves is to engage in individual therapy and/or support groups. Individual therapy, during which the caregivers can develop a trusting relationship with the therapist, allows caregivers to talk about their emotions and share their burdens. In the process, caregivers may be able to gain a new perspective on their situations and in their relationship with others. Opening oneself to fresh choices about navigating through "rough waters" can be key. Individual therapy supports the health of caregivers, which in turn allows them to provide more support to their loved ones.

Support groups with other caregivers who share similar issues can be extremely helpful. The focus of the group should be explicit: will it provide informational support? Is the focus emotional support? Will the group cover both? Is the leader qualified to care for group members who might become quite emotional? Are there specific rules for group communication and maintaining privacy?

Alzheimer's has no cure, but we can heal the wounds of the diagnosis for caregivers and their partners.

You Need Help

Nobody can manage Alzheimer's caregiving alone. One way to take care of yourself is to get the help you need to provide the quality of care you want to provide. Be open to professional help—doctors, consultants, professional caregivers, etc.—and informal help from family members, friends, or volunteers. It is not only okay but *good* to hand off some of the responsibilities of caregiving to someone else to give yourself at least a little breathing room.

You know you need other people involved to get your loved one the best care. You *also* will need other people involved in order for *you* to get the self-care you need. For a lot of people, realizing they need help is an important first step.

Accept Help. If people offer to lend a hand, accept their help. In fact, keep some ideas at the ready for when someone says, "Just let me know what I can do." Because a lot of people will say that, and most will mean it, but they may never *do* anything because they don't know what would be helpful. So let them know. Say you'd love for them to come for a visit ("How's Tuesday?"), or to run an errand for you, or to come and visit with the person you care for so *you* can go out and run an errand (imagine fifteen quiet minutes in the grocery story alone).

Ask for Help. Don't be afraid to *ask* for help, even of people who haven't offered; if they offered that one time, way back, but never mentioned it again; or if they helped you another time, but you could use help again. Friends and family won't always offer, but most will be glad to know, specifically, how they can help. This goes for official caregivers as well: tell them what you want and need from their work. If you don't explain that you want them to play games or put on music, rather than put on the TV, they might not know. Asking for help is *not* failing; it is coping effectively with the harsh realities of the disease.

Help Yourself. Just remember, it is okay to ask for help in order to do something that is about *you*. Ask a friend to hold down the fort so that you can go to the gym or get your nails done so you can feel human again. Don't go it alone. Let others do for you, at least some of the time.

Your Attitude Matters

Jill Smith at Byrd Institute says she likes Michael's and my "it-is-what-it-is" attitude. It's not something she sees every day. But it goes right along with our 24-Hour Rule: you've got a day to process whatever has happened, particularly anything negative, but then you move on. Life gives you lemons; you make lemonade. I don't want to minimize the magnitude of what people with Alzheimer's, and their caregivers, are facing. But dwelling on the negatives doesn't do anyone any good. There's no point in wallowing. Or in freaking out all the time. Michael and I are glass-half-full—and overflowing—kinds of people.

Your attitude in all this matters—to the person with Alzheimer's, to the kind of care you can give, and to the way *you* feel—physically, emotionally, and spiritually. Our attitudes are multifaceted. No one is going to be excellent at everything, all the time. Let's just agree that you'll cut yourself a break when you ask yourself how you're doing as a caregiver. Here are a few things that can help: acceptance, sense of humor, patience, and realism.

Aim for Acceptance

This book is about the things you can do to improve your situation. The truth is, though, that much about this disease and all it brings in its wake cannot be changed. In those cases, I aim for acceptance. I don't have to like it, but if I can't change it, why waste my time and energy on it? It is what it is, so I move on.

Have a Sense of Humor

A sense of humor is important in facing change and uncertainty. The ability to maintain your sense of humor and find ways to laugh often will power you through this journey. You are facing something deadly serious, but try not to take *yourself* too seriously. Keep a light touch. Joking around is one way to take some of the sting out of a situation and to reduce its power over you. What could defeat a person who literally laughs in the face of Alzheimer's?

Your humor may be a little dark, but so what? Years ago, when we were sitting in Dr. Yucus's office during our initial discovery of Michael's diagnosis, I noticed the mood was somber. We needed a little levity. I looked straight across the desk and said, "So you're telling me my husband has CRS disease?" I could tell by the look on his face that he didn't know what I meant, so I reiterated: "<u>C</u>an't <u>R</u>emember <u>S</u>hit disease?" Even at that moment, we needed some humor, something I use every single day.

Find Patience

Alzheimer's is frustrating in so many ways, so maintaining patience is especially challenging. But to care for a person with Alzheimer's, you are definitely going to need a lifetime supply of patience in a concentrated period of time. This will help you keep things in perspective and continue to move forward. However, forgiving yourself when you lose your patience (and you will) is equally important.

Be Realistic

Keep your expectations of yourself (and the person you are caring for) in check. Do what you can to the best of your ability. Know your limits. Keep trying. This is real life; nothing about it is going to be perfect.

Surround Yourself with Positive People

One of the best things you can do is to surround yourself with positive people. Choose friends and family who will be there for you. You'll want to be around empathetic, supportive individuals who have patience and understanding (or the desire to acquire understanding)—people who make you feel better.

On the flip side: don't waste your time and energy on people who are not lifting you up. Alzheimer's caregiving is tough enough as it is; you don't need anyone else's negative energy bringing you down. You can't afford relationships with people who are judgmental or undermining. As for those who withdraw or don't want to be bothered, allow yourself to let go, at least for the time being.

That said, try to cut people some slack. A few may be afraid, in denial, uninformed, or simply unsure how to conduct themselves around a person with Alzheimer's. A lot of people without their own direct experience with the disease are just not good at "getting" what you are going through. The truth is people say stupid things. Even well-meaning people do this. The only thing you can control is your response, so don't let it get to you. Letting it get to you is not going to help anything or anyone. Unfortunately, some people may disappoint you, so be sure to remember your 24-Hour Rule—let it go, continue to surround yourself with positive and supportive people, and leave the others on the sidelines. I affectionately call it a permanent time-out.

Some gentle coaching can help, which may shift the relationship back into a positive mode. Always leave the door open, make specific suggestions to those who are open to them, and then keep what works for you and let go of what doesn't.

What's good for the person you're caring for—eating well, establishing a routine, planning for the future, socializing—is usually good for you too. The inverse applies as well: what's good for you is good for the other person. Even if it means leaving for a while when your loved one doesn't want you to go; even if the person who steps in to help in your absence doesn't do things exactly the way you do. Taking a break may cost money (within the realm of what you can afford) and take energy to arrange. But it's worth it, because this is a long road, and your health and happiness are vital to everyone involved.

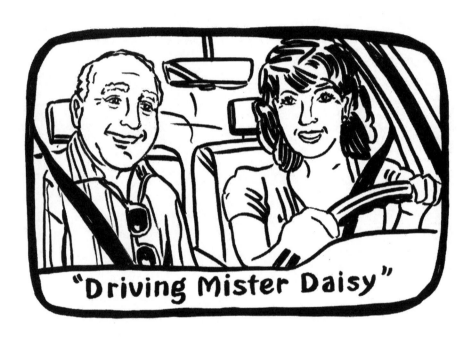

CHAPTER 11

DECISIONS ABOUT DRIVING

I think the hardest part of Michael's diagnosis occurred when the doctor told him he should not drive anymore. This seemed more difficult to accept than being told he had to stop working. At least the latter could be considered early retirement, something more readily accepted in our culture. In both cases, it wasn't his choice, and that hurt. No one ever wants to give up driving.

But for someone with Alzheimer's, driving is a safety issue and therefore he had no choice. Once a driver is disoriented or lost, it's not unusual for his or her driving to worsen. You might not recognize some of the other issues as easily. For example, spatial perception weakens, which makes it harder to stay in the correct lane. An individual with Alzheimer's may also become confused when it's time to turn right or left, and may neglect to properly signal. A person may become overwhelmed by the sheer amount of stimuli that accompanies driving—all the noise, visuals whizzing by, and so on. It's common to turn into a very nervous driver, always afraid someone is about to turn into your lane or fail to brake. Feeling out of control behind the wheel of a car is nerve-racking and unsafe for *anyone*.

People with Alzheimer's who drive put themselves and others at risk, making the situation a public safety issue. We want to protect our loved ones from hurting themselves *and* others.

Maybe handing over the keys doesn't happen on day one, but it is definitely going to be necessary. It's never going to be an easy adjustment, but once you are in a "new normal," the person with Alzheimer's will become accustomed to new ways of getting around. Plus, the caregiver no longer has to worry about his or her loved one's safety.

For Michael and me, we try to take a light touch on this tough subject. For example, when I'm at the wheel, or Michael is catching a ride with Lee or someone else, we say he's being "Mr. Daisy," a reference to the 1989 movie *Driving Miss Daisy*. This way, Michael avoids wallowing in the loss of his driver's license and, instead, can enjoy being chauffeured around.

What If Someone Does Not Want to Give Up Driving?

Thank goodness Michael came around to trading his driver's license for a generic state photo ID—sort of a non-driver's license—without too much drama, a perfect example of the 24-Hour Rule in action. But it's common for people with Alzheimer's to put up quite a fight on this topic. You can't really blame them: you wouldn't want to lose this freedom either. But you simply have to figure out a way to make it happen.

Julie Fohrman, a gerontologist and geriatric care manager here in the Chicago area, walked me through the options if you find yourself in that position. (Actually, Julie has walked me through a *lot* of stuff about safety for Alzheimer's, and I'm really sorry that I didn't start to work with her years earlier; it would have saved me a lot of time and effort.) Consider these:

- Hospitals, rehab centers, and senior centers often offer driving safety evaluations sponsored with the DMV, and they may be covered under Medicare. Or check with a physical or occupational therapist. Hearing and vision screening also might be good yardsticks. Sometimes having objective measures that indicate the time to stop driving has come makes it easier to accept.
- Investigate alternate forms of transportation. Let the person who needs to stop driving know that it doesn't mean he or she won't be able to get around. For example, options may be available for walking or biking. And explain the degree to which you (or other friends, family members, or caregivers) will be available as a driver. Beyond that, present information on taxis, senior center vans, and services staffed by volunteers that take people to doctor's appointments. Uber and other ride and ride-sharing services have been a great addition to this kind of list, where they are available. (I love the way Uber lets you to rate your driver, and leave comments.)
- Demonstrate the affordability of these alternatives. Some people end up saving money when they stop driving. Plus, you may be able to get financial help like cab vouchers. You can calculate how much money will be saved on gas and insurance (and car payments, if relevant) too. If a person's car is sold, that money can be "banked"—literally or symbolically—to

cover other transportation costs. Some people find financial discussions like these especially convincing.
- One more financial argument: with a diagnosis of Alzheimer's, a person can no longer get auto insurance. In some states, doctors are required to report the diagnosis to the health department, which will notify the DMV. Even if doctors are not required to do this, and you don't tell your insurance company yourself, if you do have an accident, the investigation will uncover the diagnosis and your policy won't pay out. The risk a person takes driving with Alzheimer's is not just to life and limb, but also to financial security.
- Ask the person's doctor for help. Not all doctors will be willing to get involved in talking to people about the need to stop driving, but many will. The expert opinion of a trusted authority is what some people need to get them to make this transition. Doctors can provide referrals to driver evaluation programs, as mentioned above. A physician can even file with the DMV to revoke someone's license.
- Report the person to the DMV yourself. (Sometimes the way to do this is to go through the police department and notify them of an impaired driver.) There should then be a letter that comes to the person at home, asking the individual to come in to the DMV for driver safety testing.
- If necessary, hide, disable, give away, or sell the car. Maybe your neighbor has an extra spot in his garage? Some people might be persuaded to give the car to someone who needs it, perhaps as a permanent loan—or gift—to a child or grandchild. Though it may feel uncomfortable resorting to these

extreme measures, remember that you must do everything you can to keep your loved one—and the rest of the drivers on the road—safe.

Take the Test

I urge everyone to take the driving evaluation test available through hospitals and rehab facilities. There's a two-part test—a written portion and a drive using a simulator—and if you pass those you get taken out in an actual car with an evaluator. Here's what you should know about this: you can choose the area in which you take the test. The first time Michael took it, they had him drive around the hospital, an area where he had never driven. When he failed that, we agreed to have him take it again in our neighborhood.

As it turns out, the evaluator will pick you up at your home. This makes sense to me, since most people taking this sort of test are avoiding difficult routes, especially those within high speed limits. Like Michael, they are probably more comfortable limiting their driving to easier trips, like out to the store and back, or just over to the golf course, or the coffee shop. Also, note that it's best to take a test drive where you're more likely to travel.

Michael didn't pass the second test, but driving locally defused a lot of the tension. And I think we were both able to accept the results more readily, because he was at least set up to succeed. Plus, the familiar streets around our house meant no crowds, waiting in line, or all that accompanies a test originating at a hospital or the DMV.

Turning in the License

Here's something I wish I'd known before Michael and I went through it: the DMV has to literally destroy your license when you turn it in. And at least here, they have you witness it. I suppose that is reassuring to some people—the license won't be floating around out there waiting for someone to use it to steal your identity—but in point of fact they don't *have* to do it right in front of you. That moment was incredibly difficult. If I could go back in time I'd call ahead to find someone who could help arrange for us to surrender the license peacefully and avoid watching it be destroyed.

CHAPTER 12

LOOKING AND FEELING GOOD

This illness threatens to rob people of their dignity. It happens in so many ways, but maintaining personal hygiene is one the best ways to help people with Alzheimer's keep their dignity. Still, taking care of your own body gets complicated with an Alzheimer's diagnosis. People might forget to brush their teeth or take a shower or forget *how*. Figuring out how to guide and support these basic routines and habits has a big payoff. Both you and your loved one avoid embarrassment. Some personal hygiene measures also are necessary to maintain good health. Taking care of things as you always have is a good way to connect to "normal" life and sustain a daily routine. It's also crucial for self-esteem. And don't think for a minute that helping someone with Alzheimer's maintain a nice appearance is superficial; it's a meaningful and important way to help this person navigate the disease.

The Power of a Compliment
Sometimes—and I'm just being honest—I've wanted to say, "Whew! Honey, your breath!" or "Sweetheart, you're looking rather scraggly today." But it's true what they say about catching more flies with honey, and I pour it on: "Hey handsome, will you shave for

me? I love the feel of your smooth face." Or "Look at those pearly whites flash—you have such a great smile." Caring messages like these are good for the relationship in general, but with regard to hygiene these phrases are simply more helpful. In many cases, your loved one is less likely to be defensive or embarrassed. I think it helps people engage with the process of taking care of themselves, and engaging is always good. So, whenever possible, I emphasize the positive rather than call attention to the negative.

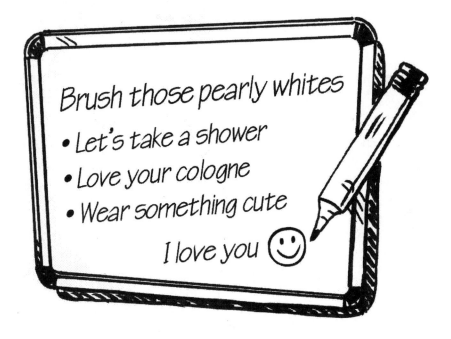

Another Reason We Cannot Do Without a Whiteboard
You already know how much we depend on an erasable whiteboard to manage our day. This is especially true with regard to the one in

our bathroom, which Michael sees every day before heading down to the kitchen. I fill it out first thing every morning, before I go downstairs. It's like the classic note-on-the-mirror, only with room for more information.

The basic messages are mostly the same each day, but I add cute notes to keep it fresh, friendly, and attention getting. So it's a little step up from just a boring list: "Please shave," next to a smiley face. Or I'll write, "Remember to brush, XO," and "How about a little of that cologne I love?" I also use it to call out anything special about the day that might affect morning preparations—"You're golfing today—dress casual."

Do It Together

If you can, check these must-do items off the list with your loved one. Doing so keeps it more casual. In fact, you might write something like "Let's go brush our teeth before we go out" instead of "Go brush your teeth." That way the item seems less like an annoying reminder and more like just another activity you can accomplish as a team.

Admittedly, this next tip won't be right for everybody, but for us the "do it together" approach is great for showers too. For us, this can occasionally be a romantic moment—we have to take those where we can. But other times it's just a get-it-done thing, more or less like brushing teeth at the same time. And sometimes it's just a way to avoid a tougher conversation about what is and isn't being done. That's a real part of our life now, but it's not a topic we have to address every day.

Sometimes we are not literally doing things at the same time, but still take a "we're-in-this-together" approach. For example, I might say, "Honey, you shower first since I take longer." It's a reminder, disguised as just a bit of logistics. Put this way, it's clear that we both need to take showers, even if we're taking turns.

Make It an Event

My favorite approach to what could be a boring subject is to make personal grooming into a fun activity. For example, Michael and I now go for mani/pedis together. True, I pick brighter shades of nail polish, and he may be in it only for the foot massage, but we both end up with tidy nails *and* a little "couple time." We go the a nail salon, but you can easily make your own event at home as long as you really sell it, with nice-smelling cream massaged into hands and a warm-water soak before trimming. Like so much about Alzheimer's care—and life in general—your attitude is key.

Haircuts are another good opportunity to turn something from your to-do list into an outing. Pick the right salon, talk to the hairdressers in advance if necessary, see if you can get seated side by side, and, if the staff offers you any small luxuries—Tea while you wait? *People* magazine?—say, "Yes!"

But remember, before you turn something into a special event, consider your loved one's comfort zone, which, with Alzheimer's, is a moving target. For example, someone might have a strong preference for what's familiar, so choosing a new place to get a haircut may not be a good idea. On the other hand, you might discover that a new activity holds appeal—Michael in the pedicure chair being a prime example.

Personal grooming is good for: maintaining general hygiene, staying connected to everyday life, having successful social interactions, and reinforcing self-esteem and independence. You can even reap other rewards like a personal bonding experience, a relaxing or adventurous time, and a form of self-expression. Little things can make a big difference.

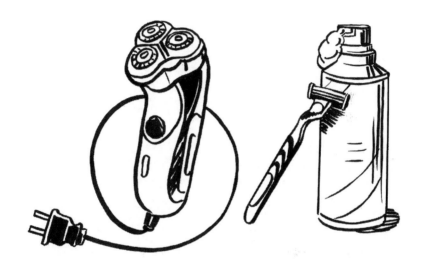

Play It Safe

As with everything else, you'll want to keep one eye on safety even when you're dealing with something as ordinary as personal hygiene. For example, Michael switched from a regular razor blade to an electric razor. You'll want to make sure products are very clearly labeled—you won't want to mix up tubes of hair gel and toothpaste. Similarly, only necessary items should be left easily accessible. Maybe you don't need the hair gel on the counter at all, and the nail scissors should live in the closet now, not in that little dish right next to the sink.

One other way I "play it safe" is to double-check that important hygiene items have actually been completed. For example, unless I am with Michael when he brushes his teeth, I will take a look at his toothbrush before bed to make sure it has actually been used. Maybe skipping a day poses no immediate risk, but skip too many days and you could be looking at a dental disaster.

Getting Dressed

Dressing turns out to be harder than you might think. That's because it's actually quite a complex task, or set of tasks, requiring many different skills at once. It's common for Alzheimer's to interfere with one or more of these skills. Getting dressed is complicated physically (buttoning buttons, tying a tie) and mentally (What's appropriate for today's weather? What do I need to be ready for today's activity?). At each step, your loved one might forget how and in what order to dress. And if coordination is an issue, that could make the process even more difficult and frustrating.

So my best advice is to simplify as much as possible: pull-on pants, no-button shirts, limited color palette (so nothing clashes), and so forth. Michael likes to wear the same things over and over; he likes what's familiar, and comfortable, so I get multiples of favorite items. Also, leave plenty of time to avoid dressing in a rush.

Like everything else in our new normal, my goal is for Michael to handle getting dressed as independently as possible. For example,

I'll offer guidance by announcing that it's time to get ready to go to the gym, then encourage him to go upstairs and get dressed in workout clothes. Or we might go into the closet together and I'll say "How about that blue sweatshirt with those jeans? You look so cute in that outfit." Or something like, "Weather report says it's going to be cold all day, so you might want a sweater over that." I'm not issuing a command, nor do I sound too nitpicky. And, yes, you may have noticed some familiar themes: use compliments, and do it together.

Keep It Clean

Keeping clean and dirty clothes separate can be a real challenge in our house (though I think it is fairly common). For example, Michael tends to pull off a shirt, fold it, and return it to the shelf. He doesn't remember doing that, so the next day he'll pull it out and wear it again. To avoid this, I make a mental note each day of what he's wearing, then I go into the closet and take out what should go into the laundry instead. Most of the time we change together anyway—"Let's go get into our sweats," I'll say—so I'm right there to redirect clothes as necessary.

The best plan is to make a system you both can follow. Whatever gets accomplished on a day-to-day basis in the same way has the best chance of getting done. Right now, the closet strategy isn't working so well, but we're making great strides emptying Michael's gym bag. When he comes home from the gym, he always removes his clothes from the bag and puts them in the hamper. It has become a regular routine.

Shoes

Some people think of shoes as part of getting dressed, but I've had to do enough problem-solving around the issue of footwear that I'm giving it a paragraph all its own. We went through a phase when Michael would never take off his shoes. He even wore them to bed. Finally, I realized that his reluctance to remove his shoes had everything to do with his desire never to have to put them on again. He'd forgotten how to do it and, understandably, didn't want to ask for help, underscoring the importance of tuning in to the people we're caring for, watching what they do, listening to what they say, and generally figuring out where they are coming from. Only then can we think creatively about workarounds and solutions. In this particular case, if I didn't want to sleep with tennis shoes in my bed, we had to get Michael footwear he felt confident he could manage.

Losing the laces is one the first strategies we adopted. Take it from me: they're definitely not worth the trouble. Initially, we used Velcro, but even that became too much of a challenge, and when that occurs it's time to create a new plan. Now, Michael wears gym shoes designed with drawstrings. Other than those, he wears shoes that slip on easily and stay on securely.

Manage Frustration

I've said it before, and I'll say it again: you can't get frustrated when things go awry. You'll get worked up, your loved one will follow your lead, and nothing will improve. So if Michael puts on multiple shirts, or something winds up backward, or he doesn't realize he's mixed something up, I'll just leave it alone if we're not going out anywhere. If it seems like a planned activity will go more smoothly if we have a little intervention before we leave the house, then I'll try the old, "That's a great shirt, such a good color on you, but I think it's got a stain . . . " or "It's going up to 85 today, so I think you'll be glad if you get rid of some of those layers." I try to be as straightforward and kind as possible. Sometimes playful works better, so I'll say, "Uh-oh, better start over" and, at the same time, sneak in a hug and a kiss while changing. The idea is to defuse the situation so the other person does not get frustrated.

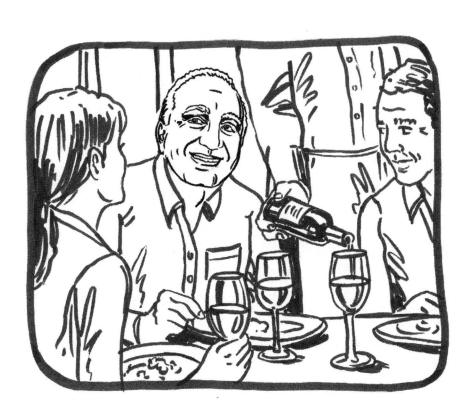

CHAPTER 13

BE INTERACTIVE

With Michael's early retirement, we experienced many changes. He asked himself all sorts of difficult questions, like, "Who am I when I am not working?" and "What do I do with my time now?" I asked, "Who is he going to hang out with?"

Michael and I have always been a very social couple, spending lots of time with friends. We're *people* people. Michael is used to going out to do "guy stuff," like golfing or tennis or just going out for a beer. For us, staying socially active is important for maintaining a normal routine *and* for brain health. But Michael's friends were mostly men in their fifties, and they worked all day. So I knew we would need to become more intentional about arranging a social life in our new normal.

So we decided to look for a "buddy" for Michael (see Chapter 5: Finding a "Buddy"). At the time I had a job, so this provided Michael guy time while I worked during the day. I've since retired and, aside from hanging out with me, Michael's relationship with Lee has provided a steady and fulfilling opportunity for socializing. Our time with family and friends is equally important, even when the logistics for getting together take some extra effort. I make it a point to stay connected, reaching out to friends and family, making regular social plans, and planning weekend visits. For Michael and me, engaging in fun, enjoyable activities with other active people is a part of our life and history together. Now this is even more important, since it helps stimulate the brain, which is always good. Plus, it significantly adds to our quality of life. Our new normal wouldn't be good—or normal—without it.

Ken D'Agostino, Longtime Friend

When Michael is engaged, he's a marvelous friend. I find it easy to have a conversation with Michael, frequently about the old days when we worked together. I keep it general, not too specific, and we talk about our real estate days. Some days I'll say something to him and I can see he doesn't understand, so I back off. Why would I push? I'll find something else to talk about, because there is no reason whatsoever to make it hard for him. If he's losing a word, I can gently help him find it. I try not to talk faster than he can absorb so he doesn't lose the thread of the conversation.

My philosophy is the same I've always used in business. In real estate, you have to be good at listening to and connecting with all kinds of people—and that is to appreciate the level of whoever you are talking to, and meet the person there. That's the same for everybody, so of course it's the way I interact with Michael. I don't think that's magical—to give him the grace of living at his speed.

The Right Environment

Socializing successfully means choosing the right environment to make sure Michael feels secure. We have to create opportunities to interact with those people who make him feel comfortable. Determining the right environment can be challenging. As with everything else, we keeping learning and adjusting. When planning a social occasion, I focus on:

- Noise level: I look for quiet, pleasant surroundings, which may mean making dinner reservations early, before crowds make a lovely place noisy. Too much background clatter makes it more difficult to follow conversations.
- Group size: Large groups don't work well for us. Going out with two other people is usually best, and maybe up to six people at the most.
- Seating arrangements: When Michael and I go out to eat, we always sit side by side, with Michael on the inside if the table is next to a wall. Reducing distractions makes it easier for him to stay engaged in a conversation; he's less likely to disconnect. If we are out with a group of six people, I always ask for a round table because that facilitates one conversation among everyone rather than multiple side conversations.
- Timing: Avoid peak times at any venue or event. We often leave early from long or loud events. Better to leave while it is still fun than to push it too long and end up overtired and frustrated. In other words, exit on a high note.
- Placement: If we are at an event with a lot of people (family wedding, for example), we "work the room" from the perimeter. Plunging into the middle of the room and the center of the action, which used to be our MO, is too overwhelming. Even though large groups can be difficult, Michael is

always comfortable at family functions and when surrounded by good friends.

The Road Not Taken

Thanks to a large network of family and friends, and the good fortune of finding Michael's "buddy," Lee, we continue to enjoy an active social life, and I feel confident Michael is reaping the benefits socializing brings. We continue to surround ourselves with people who support us and understand our limitations. This is key to a successful social environment for Michael.

For us, this has provided ample social opportunities. You can mix it up by checking out other venues. Community centers usually offer programs for seniors and a range of other classes, workshops, and trips that provide opportunities for socializing. Adult day care centers for people with Alzheimer's are another way to go but may be more appropriate for people in more advanced stages of the disease. Sometimes the socializing opportunities are an important factor in choosing that residential care. Support groups, too, are especially advantageous for people in the early stages of Alzheimer's.

Eating Out

Socializing for us most often means going out for a nice meal. Here are some strategies that help all those brunches, lunches, and dinners go smoothly:

Help in ordering. You might have taken ordering off a menu—especially one with many choices—for granted, but this can become an overwhelming task for someone with Alzheimer's. A person might also forget what it is, exactly, that they really like to eat. It's not uncommon for people with Alzheimer's to order what they hear around them by simply repeating what they've heard, whether they like the dish or not.

All of this can create stress. Luckily, this is an easy problem to defuse. Sometimes I go through the menu with Michael and highlight a couple choices for him. I often suggest a couple general choices ("Do you want chicken or the fish tonight?") or offer a recommendation. For example, I might say, "I heard the grilled salmon is really good here. Would you like that?" Or I suggest splitting something and say, "I can't decide between the chicken Vesuvio and the grilled salmon. Do you want to share?"

Mind your manners. Some social niceties begin to slip after an Alzheimer's diagnosis. Your job then is to gently help your loved one do what's conventionally expected without calling attention to the omission. For example, if Michael has forgotten to put a napkin in his lap, I might just do it for him without saying a word. Or I might remind him as I'm doing the same thing so it doesn't seem like a big deal. That helps him *see* what I'm doing, which can augment his comprehension. Sometimes Michael uses the "wrong" utensil. I generally let it go if his technique is getting the job done. Who cares if he's eating chopped salad with a spoon rather than a fork? But if it's causing an avoidable challenge, I point that out casually, and offer an alternative: "Maybe try this fork: it might be easier."

Reservations. I always call the restaurant in advance to explain our special requests (quiet or round table, etc.), and they are almost always accommodating when I explain. (I've said it before and I'll say it again: tell everyone; Alzheimer's is not a secret.) By now, all our favorite spots know Michael and everyone does his or her best to create an enjoyable experience for us both.

Manage the conversation. The most important rule for successful socializing is to let everyone know what works best. Following a conversation can be difficult for people with Alzheimer's, but including them and keeping them engaged is essential—and it's easy. Still, you'll need to help others understand both the limitations and what works best. Some people may know intuitively what to do, but many feel put off if they aren't sure how to handle themselves, so sharing what you know will work is always a good idea.

When dining out, or in small groups, try to avoid conversations in which people are speaking too quickly and louder than necessary. And stick to one conversation at a time. Cross talk is confusing, whether it's happening next to your loved one or across the table. Keeping the group focused on one conversation all together also will help a person with Alzheimer's stay engaged. You may need to do a little maneuvering to include the person in a group conversation; jumping in solo can be difficult. You may address a particular question to your loved one with a good opening. Sometimes I feed Michael a line because getting started can be the hardest part. So if the group is talking business, I might say something like, "Michael, I think you were saying earlier that you don't trust this market to last." He might pick up that theme (*you* try to stop Michael from sharing his opinions on the stock market or politics . . .), and even if he acknowledges me with a simple "Yes," he's at least in the game.

Andrea Saewitz, Longtime Friend
My husband and I have been friends with Cheryl and Michael for a very long time now. I can't be down on people who are scared or

uncomfortable about someone with Alzheimer's, but you just have to try to see past it. That may not always be easy to do, but it is with Michael. He's a sweet guy, always has been. He's an easy guy to love.

Cheryl helped us from the beginning, explaining what Michael's needs were as his mind was changing, giving us tips like being sure to look him in the face, keep distractions to a minimum, repeating things as necessary. It won't be obvious, but sometimes Cheryl will cajole him for a comment, or ask him, "What do you think?" and even provide answers for him.

My husband and I make a real point of including him in the conversation, making sure he is engaged. I always greet him with "It's Andrea!" so he doesn't have to be at a loss. When all is said and done, you just have to be a little more sensitive.

Reach Out

This can be hard for caregivers to accept, but some people are going to pull away from a person with Alzheimer's. This disease can make others uncomfortable. It's too scary. Or they simply don't know how to act. In some cases, it's too sad to see someone who seems so dramatically different from the person they've known. A day without reaching out to connect becomes a week, which turns into a month, and then six months. Eventually, you realize that the person who used to be a friend has stopped calling to make plans or even just to say hello. I have learned to accept the disappointment. Now I move toward and surround myself with the people who continue to show their love and support.

When a person pulls away, it is much more hurtful to the caregiver, who understands that the relationship is over. Unfortunately, the person with Alzheimer's doesn't understand or feel that rejection. So carefully choose the people with whom you want to socialize. Continue making social plans with positive people. If someone is going to be negative rather than positive, you don't need that in your life now anyway.

On the other hand, you will also find that, in your new normal, some people become closer; you may discover you have support in unlikely places.

Still, you probably want to reach out to others, even the ones who can't bring themselves to reach out to you. I try to give everyone the benefit of the doubt, but with some people there will come a time when you have to say enough is enough and move on. Life is too precious and time is even more precious, so be selective and honest with yourself. Before you get to the point of dropping friends, it may help to give people some coaching on how best to interact. For example, suggest that they introduce themselves each time, specifying their connection: "Michael, it's your old friend Ken . . ." This avoids potential embarrassment and awkwardness all around.

Another specific strategy that has worked well for us is posting lots of photos on Facebook so that everyone can see how active Michael is, how he enjoys being with friends and family. The smile on his face in these pictures—at graduations, on weekend trips, and out for dinners—is unmistakable.

One more thing: now is a great time to let the past stay in the past. Whatever bad blood may have happened in the past, reach out to family and friends and make a connection with those who want to respond. And if anyone reaches out to you despite problems in the past, consider creating a new relationship.

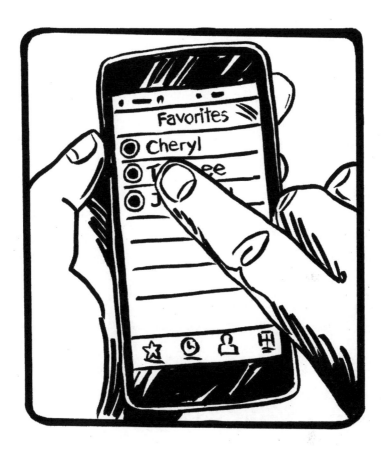

Please Call Again

The phone is an important tool for keeping a person with Alzheimer's in touch with family and friends, but it comes with complications of its own. It can be harder to converse over the phone than in person. Without visuals to provide clues to meaning and emotion, it's difficult to maintain focus. And technology has its challenges. Placing a call has become hard for Michael, and knowing how to answer a call even harder. All of this makes it challenging for family and friends who live out of town. So I help to make it easier for Michael to stay connected.

On top of all that, a lot of people are hesitant to call. I've learned that many are uncomfortable trying to help Michael get through a telephone conversation. I try to explain what they may not see: Michael doesn't realize it's awkward. For him, it's just a plain pleasure to hear from people. I encourage them to not stress over unanswered questions or long pauses or non sequiturs. "Just roll with it," I say. I also recommend that people avoid asking open-ended questions; it's too hard for someone with Alzheimer's to process and answer in a timely fashion.

However the call goes, the basic message—"I called because I care about you" or "I'm thinking of you"—always comes through. I ask them not to get discouraged, because getting a call always puts a smile on Michael's face. Also, I ask that people do not leave messages, since he doesn't know how to retrieve them. When I explain it's better to just try again another time, most people are willing to shift their phone habits and accommodate my request.

I also explain that Michael can't call them. It's not that he doesn't want to talk; he's simply forgotten how to make that happen. I suggest they call my cell and then I can hand the phone to Michael with a quick mention of who's calling and why: "Honey, it's Bryan calling just to say 'hi.'" I hope that when I explain how much Michael enjoys these calls, people will continue to connect. Unfortunately, that's not foolproof, so I often place a call myself and then hand the phone over to Michael. Or I might reach out to friends, especially if Michael is a little down, and specifically ask them to reach out, explaining how helpful this will be. I usually call Michael's close friends, Bryan Fields and Ken D'Agostino, because both, without fail, will call when Michael needs it most. I am so grateful for those special friends.

Being Together

Our neurologist, Dr. Chad Yucus, emphasized to us early on the importance of social interaction. As he put it: "Isolation precipitates functional and cognitive decline." The research supports this. A study published in the *Archive of General Psychiatry* concluded that lonely people had *twice* the risk of the disease. That article pointed out that both *being* alone—having few social interactions—and *feeling* alone (regardless of how many interactions you have) are risk factors. I think the socializing in Michael's life is providing help to slow down the progression of the disease, so I do all I can to keep Michael in regular interaction with a range of positive people.

In our "new normal," I've had to think carefully about how we socialize. But in the big picture, I recommend one strategy in particular: enjoy each other and your time together.

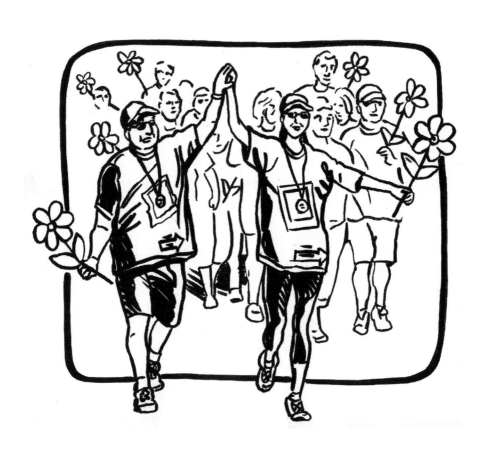

CHAPTER 14

CHAMPIONING YOUR LOVED ONE

After Michael's diagnosis, I started talking about Alzheimer's to everyone, mostly to garner support. But over time I discovered that by discussing the disease, all of us—my friends, family, and strangers too—were helping to raise awareness, erase the stigma associated with the disease, and increase support for Alzheimer's causes.

Michael and I are open with each other as well. Many people with Alzheimer's feel powerless. Even the strongest and smartest people want to live in denial. Some don't even realize when they are in denial. We chose to face it head on, together, and with the wider world. This has empowered and propelled us to move forward.

Talk It Up

The first instinct for some people who receive an Alzheimer's diagnosis is to wall themselves off from family and friends. A toxic and heartbreaking combination of fear, embarrassment, and even shame are at work in that decision. But nothing good can come of isolation. We've discussed Michael's condition with our family, friends, and colleagues. Plus, I've become well known for telling people all about the disease just in the course of our everyday lives. I believe in letting people know there's an issue and how they can help. This is one of the most important ways to advocate for your loved one and help yourself in the process.

Most people want to be supportive, but many don't know how. They have neither the tools nor the experience. Still, a little communication goes a long way. Most people step up, which is especially true for people *not* intimately connected to you. In these small, ordinary ways, you are creating real change in the world—raising awareness, increasing sensitivity, and putting others in a position to be supportive.

Early on in our "new normal" lifestyle, Michael and I took a once-in-a-lifetime bike trip through Italy with the wonderful B&R tour company. Filling out the paperwork, I made sure to let them know about Michael's situation and how it might impact the tour. Mostly, though, I wanted to make sure the tour would be appropriate for us. I also wanted to give the company a heads up to minimize uncomfortable and embarrassing moments, which can arise if people are not aware of the disease and its impact. I also wanted to make sure we could avoid any safety hazards along the way.

Then something truly special took place three days into the trip, which just so happened to be our anniversary. In the words of our guide Irena:

Improvising with the few resources available, we used everything we could think of, even decorating with toilet paper, to create the perfect ambiance. As everyone arrived for what they thought was the start of just another day riding through the Tuscan countryside, the courtyard was decorated with streaming white, the aisles of bikes were set up like pews, and my co-guide and I awaited Cheryl and Michael at the "altar" (table for ride snacks and sunscreen). Wearing our bathrobes!

The happy couple repeated special vows made just for them, including lines like "I place this Torroncino ring upon your finger, as a symbol of my eternal friendship, that I will always stay on the right side of the road, and slow down when you are not near me."

As they walked out the gates, we threw rice, popped champagne, and waved as the happy couple rode off on their bikes for a cruise through Tuscany.

I'm telling you this story 1) because you will see why I called B&R "wonderful," and 2) because this is why I tell *everyone* about Alzheimer's and its role in our life. When people understand your situation, they can offer support above and beyond your expectations. Or, to put it another way, when you withhold the truth of your situation, you are robbing other people of the opportunity to show kindness—something other people genuinely want to do. Here's Irena again: *"As we learned quickly, Cheryl did not like to stray far from Michael. Her compassion and deep care for him were easily apparent. I was very touched that we could create a special moment they could always hold on to."* And hold on to it we have. Our Italy trip is a highlight of our life together and a highlight of the memory montage Michael watches almost every day.

How Can You Help Me?

When you make a routine of sharing your story with everyone you run across in daily life, people will surprise you with their kindness.

But sometimes they won't know exactly how to help, so it's up to you to get specific. Try telling:

- *The person taking reservations at a restaurant. Explain what kind of table would be useful, i.e., somewhere quiet where the whole group can comfortably hear one another. Be sure to explain why you need this, and chances are you will get what you ask for.*
- *The dentist. Anxiety levels about even just a teeth cleaning may be higher than they used to be, but with a heads up the office may be able to provide suitable supports.*
- *The people you talk to when booking travel. Depending on your specific situation, you might need preferential seating on the plane or a different way to get from point A to point B if the person you're traveling with doesn't 'do' trains.*
- *The staff at the gym. At our gym, everyone knows Michael, so there's always someone willing to run into the men's locker room to check on him or retrieve an item for me. When Michael leaves something in the locker room or on a machine, the gym calls me before I even realize the item didn't make it home.*
- *A banker. Even though I have Michael's financial power of attorney, a visit to the bank can take a long time. But I've made sure to get to know some people there, and, since they know and understand Michael, the staff accommodates our need to conduct transactions in a smooth and timely manner. Since they know us and how we handle things, I don't have to explain all over again each time we walk into the bank. This is especially important since financial and business-related issues are sensitive subjects for Michael. This is one way I—and the bank staff—can be respectful of his dignity.*

- *The pharmacy staff. You'd be amazed at how many times someone asks to talk to Michael about his medications rather than me. That doesn't work well, but we love Gena at CVS. She knows us and has helped many times, working through insurance and other issues.*

Fight Stigma

Even Michael had doubts about discussing his diagnosis with others. He worried that people would think he was crazy or stupid. Many people think Alzheimer's hits only older adults; they don't realize it can affect much younger people too. Many people are scared by Alzheimer's, as if it were contagious. And because the way our brains work is such a big part of how we define who we are, anything that impairs brain function is inherently frightening to people. Plus, most people know there's no cure for Alzheimer's and that fact alone is definitely frightening.

For all those reasons and more, I knew we had to speak up. I knew we couldn't accept this as a scarlet letter. We had to work out between ourselves, first, that it was not just okay but *necessary* to talk about this, and then whom to tell and how. Practically speaking, a lot of people have to know or, at least, should know. The more Alzheimer's is talked about, the more people understand the disease and its effects on those diagnosed. This is beneficial for individuals and communities. We hope to contribute to this process by telling our story. I have found that people are more likely to care about something when you can put a face to it.

Accentuate the Positive

Jill Smith, the director of the clinical study Michael is in at the Byrd Institute, says she thinks *not* hiding from this illness is one of the most important things Michael and I have done. We are open with each other and with everyone in our lives, and that has made a difference in Michael's progress and, hopefully, in the world as well.

Dr. Amanda Smith (no relation to Jill Smith), medical director of the Byrd study, adds that it's important to have *positive* voices addressing Alzheimer's. A lot of information is floating around about Alzheimer's, but it's rare to find a message like ours: that despite this devastating disease, we can make the most of our life together. As she put it: "Cheryl and Michael are a living testament to the fact that it is possible to live with Alzheimer's and be happy, and enjoy every day." That's how we live, and what we want to share, and we hope to inspire others with this possibility. We don't want to minimize what happens when Alzheimer's becomes a part of your world, but it is possible, and important, to appreciate the good in your life too. It's not that Alzheimer's brings goodness, but that goodness can exist in spite of it.

Participate in the "Walk to End Alzheimer's"

Being open about your story, spreading understanding of the disease, and focusing on positives are excellent ways to fight Alzheimer's, personally and societally. But getting involved in a more organized or formal way is also a great idea. Participating in an Alzheimer's Association "Walk to End Alzheimer's" is a good start. Every fall, the Alzheimer's Association sponsors 600 of these events all over the country. It's the largest event in the world dedicated to raising awareness and funds for Alzheimer's care, support, and research.

When you participate in a walk, you help the cause by raising money and educating people along the way. You also help yourself in two important ways. First, you're engaging in a purposeful, meaningful activity—the exact kind of brain stimulation you're after. (It's a great social occasion, too, especially when you create your own team to walk together.) Second, you learn in a really powerful way that *you are not alone*. Lots of people are literally walking the same walk you are, whether you are a person with a diagnosis or the caregiver. And that knowledge can provide some feeling of relief, and point the way toward support. You might know this theoretically and statistically, but when you see so many people come together, you really, instantly *know*.

Michael and I participated in our first walk early on in our "new normal." I was particularly inspired by the "Promise Garden" ceremony. All walkers receive a pinwheel flower with petals symbolizing their connection to the disease: blue for someone living with the disease, yellow for caregivers, purple for those who have lost someone to Alzheimer's, and orange for everyone else who wants to see an end to Alzheimer's. Plus, everyone walks wearing deep purple, the official color of Alzheimer's awareness.

Our team is Levin-Folio, and this year is our fourth walk. Every year we have at least fifteen or twenty people walking with us, plus Oliver and Baxter. I get chills of joy every time, looking at all the people holding flowers. It's powerful and inspiring, and continues to motivate me in my fight against Alzheimer's.

Looking out over the crowd, we see an ocean of people coming together to fight for a better future. Everyone is wearing—and holding flowers with—cheerful bright colors, which, to me, represent the kind of positive approach I want to take. People write names, intentions, or wishes on the petals of their flowers, and "plant" their flowers in a central location. It's quite a sight; you can't help but be moved by it. We've been back every year, with an ever-growing team of supporters walking with us, and an even bigger team contributing their support online.

The Walk to End Alzheimer's is a great event for everyone to experience at least once. But if making it an annual thing isn't for you, you might like to participate in other organized fundraising and awareness-raising projects. Just don't overload yourself. Do what you enjoy and find meaningful without stretching yourself too thin.

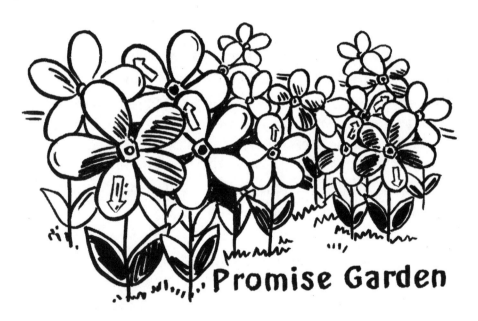

Be an Activist

We haven't gone this route yet, but for many people with Alzheimer's and their caregivers, political advocacy work is another satisfying way to engage in meaningful activity, contribute to "the cause," and get high-quality social interaction. If it's not your thing, do something else. But if it interests you, contact your local Alzheimer's Association chapter. Erna E. Colborn, President and CEO of the Greater Illinois Chapter of the Alzheimer's Association, says that many people feel empowered by bringing their personal story to politicians who can effect policy change. She also says that a lot of people, including politicians who hold the purse strings, still associate Alzheimer's only with an old woman lying in bed who can no longer speak. Erna adds that people who can present a different (and more accurate) face of Alzheimer's just by their presence make a powerful impact.

If in-person lobbying isn't your style but you want to work for change along these lines, sign up at the "Action Center" on the Alzheimer's Association website. Give them your email address, and you can receive a newsletter about Alzheimer's efforts and activities. When the Association rounds up people to sign a petition or call their member of Congress, you'll have your chance to speak up and speak out.

Erna E. Colborn, President and CEO, Alzheimer's Association, Greater Illinois Chapter

I encourage people to engage with their local Alzheimer's Association chapter. Because there is still no cure, a diagnosis can leave people feeling helpless. But getting involved, learning more about the disease, and connecting with others are quite empowering. I've seen it happen over and over and over again: people's experience changes when they learn they are not alone, that many others are facing the same issues they are, that support is available, that they don't need to be isolated, and that there are some things they can do in this fight.

When people have a brand new diagnosis, or a new realization about what they are facing, the Association offers two immediate sources of assistance. First, you can call the toll-free help line for information about the disease, caregiving, discussions families need to be having, and all the things people can do to prepare themselves quickly. The same information is available on the Association website, so people may want to explore there.

Second, schedule a meeting with our Care Navigators, who work one on one with families to begin to address difficult issues, such as what a person wants in terms of care going forward. We can help families and individuals process all the important issues that arise with this disease.

The Association covers all 50 states and Puerto Rico too. In fact, we're worldwide through our participation with Alzheimer's Disease International. If there's not a physical office easily accessible where you live, then there's a regional office just a phone call away that will offer quality information and programming in your immediate area.

Clinical Research

Another way to potentially help yourself and definitely advance knowledge of Alzheimer's in general is to volunteer as a research study subject. You may or may not be receiving the medication under study (typically, half the participants receive a placebo), and, if you get the medication, it may or may not help you (and could possibly cause side effects). But at the end of the study you'll likely have the option to participate in an extension during which you'd definitely have the opportunity to take the medication. This, too, provides invaluable information to the researchers on the longer-term efficacy of the treatment.

As I write this, Michael has just completed the 18 months of clinical trial in the study he participates in at the University of South Florida Health Byrd Alzheimer's Institute (motto: "dedicated to the prevention, treatment and cure of Alzheimer's disease and related disorders ... until Alzheimer's is a memory"). He has continued into the extension trial, which runs for another two and a half years. He's one of literally thousands of patients, but we feel very well known and cared for at the center—we know they are looking out for Michael, for us as a couple, and me as a caregiver. It was a little strange not knowing what he received during the trial, but he's had no side effects and his general ability to participate in life has been maintained even as tests show some cognitive decline. It's been a tremendous opportunity to be part of this study, and the experience has been extremely positive for both of us.

Dr. Amanda Smith, Medical Director, USF Health Byrd Alzheimer's Institute
Dr. Smith directs the study along with many others who work with her at Byrd. Her passion for caring for each individual patient, as well as advancing knowledge of and options for treating Alzheimer's, is obvious from the moment you meet her.

She is a supporter of people participating in clinical research, naturally, but also thinks it is important for people to find the right study for their situation. She emphasizes that one not sign up for a study if the stresses of participating are high. (Would it require too much time off work for the caregiver? Would repeated testing create too much anxiety?)

To participate in a study, Dr. Smith offers the following guidelines: first you have to find one, of course. Several national databases can help you in this regard, including:

- *NIH's Alzheimer's Disease Education and Referral Center (ADEAR) www.nia.nih.gov/alzheimers/clinical-trials*
- *Alzheimer's Disease Cooperative Study (ACDS) adcs.org/Studies/ClinalResearchStudy.aspx*
- *NIH's Clinicaltrials.gov clinicaltrials.gov/ct2/results?term=alzheimer%27s&Search=Search*

These can help you find a range of available options.

Step two is to determine if you are eligible for a given study. The exact criteria are specific to each study, and most are not in your control. Examples include what stage of the illness you are in, how close to the research location you live, and any other medical conditions you may have.

You will probably find you are eligible for a number of studies, so to choose where to apply you then have to weigh your preferences about what's involved in each study. Consider these factors:

- *Type of center. Is it specialized in Alzheimer's and other dementias and memory disorders, or do they do research on all types of conditions? Big academic medical centers with a specialization in Alzheimer's generally offer high levels of comprehensive*

support throughout a clinical trial. The support might not be the same at a smaller or less specialized facility, but those may be more geographically accessible and therefore more appealing.
- *Level of risk involved in relation to possible benefits and likelihood of benefit.*
- *Logistics. For example, how far will you have to travel, and how often? How long will you spend at the research center each time you go? How long does the study last?*
- *Form of treatment. Will the drug be given orally? Will you get an injection? How much cognitive testing is involved?*

This last bit of advice is from me, rather than Dr. Smith: just because you apply to a study you are eligible for doesn't mean you are going to be accepted for the study. In can be difficult to be accepted into a study, even if on paper your loved one meets all the criteria. If it is something you definitely want to do, I recommend doing whatever you can think of to make a personal connection at the research center you are applying to, like delivering your application documents in person. Help them put a face to the name, give them a chance to meet or talk to you. Every little bit helps. My personal approach is simply not to take "no" for an answer. I am Michael's true advocate in every way and remain relentless.

Tell Everyone

So much of shifting the world of Alzheimer's for the better comes down to communicating with one another. For us, it has worked wonders to tell everybody about Alzheimer's and its role in our life.

Who should you tell? Family. Friends. Neighbors. Employers. Anyone you know who may be in your situation. Anyone who knows someone who is suffering but is afraid to talk about it.

Share your story about Alzheimer's—how to understand the disease and the huge number of people affected by it. Share information about the person with Alzheimer's—personality, lifestyle, symptoms, what's helpful, and what's not. Share caregiving experiences—its stresses, its fulfilling aspects, and ways to be supportive.

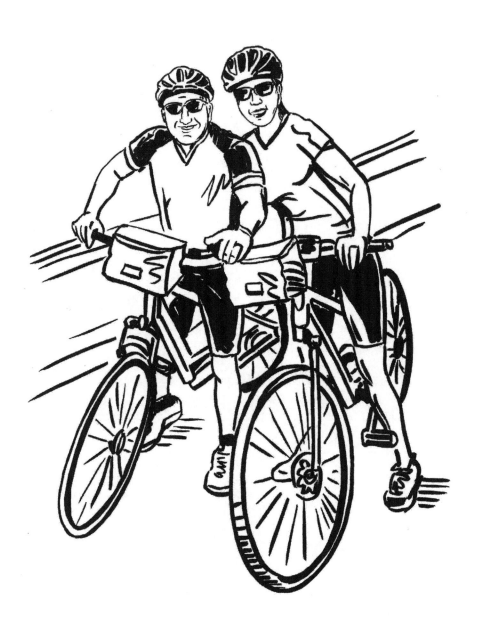

CHAPTER 15

TRAVEL SMART

Recently I took a trip with my daughter so that we could spend time together before she goes off to college in the fall. But first I flew Michael to New Jersey so that his family could step into my role. Not surprisingly, as his symptoms have progressed, travel has become more difficult for him. Still, I always try to plan a trip that is stimulating without being stressful. In the process, I've discovered that the most important part of "traveling smart" is deciding when *not* to travel.

That said, I'm a big fan of travel, and it's a love Michael and I have long shared. Even after his diagnosis, we took a lot of trips. And we still do, just not as many. Some people begin to travel *more* after a diagnosis, which I completely understand. You realize, for example, that if you're going to travel, there's never going to be a better time than the present. Travel tops the bucket list for so many people, and as long as you travel smart, I say go for it.

Michael and I went on the trip of a lifetime about two years after his diagnosis. We biked all over Italy with a small group, expert guides, and a bit of careful planning. Even with a different hotel every day, Michael did extremely well. We had a wonderful time and shared an amazing experience. And I'm glad we did it when we did for so many reasons. Taking the same trip today would not be possible.

Know Before You Go
Here's what to think about before you decide to go anywhere:

- What are the benefits of this trip to the person with Alzheimer's? Make sure you are realistic in answering this question.
- What are the challenges likely to be? Are there any ways to avoid or minimize them? Do the upsides outweigh the downsides?
- Are you okay with handling all the planning, preparation, and execution on your own? Can you manage the itineraries, confirmations, luggage, and other necessary details?

Your niece's wedding three states away is sure to be lovely, and you really want to catch up with those second cousins, and at another time maybe you and your loved one would both jump at the chance for a live band and an open bar. But for some people this is a setup for serious anxiety and discomfort, with too much noise, too much disruption to routine, and too many unfamiliar faces. Or maybe your loved one has always been particularly close with this branch of the family, and if you can drive instead of fly, and get a quiet table at the back of the reception, all will go smoothly. The important piece here is to take your best guess *before* you commit to a trip.

Choosing and Planning a Successful Trip
Carefully choosing and planning the right trip are the keys to success. You have to know the limitations of your situation, even though that is a moving target. Understand where you are and what that

might mean for travel situations. Choosing the right environment is critical. Arranging as much as you can in your favor—ahead of time—makes everything easier once you are away from home. Here are some additional strategies to consider:

- Simplify your itinerary. Don't try to pack too much in—to the trip as a whole or any given part. Pace yourself. Allow plenty of time for each activity. Schedule times to rest, and include some downtime in each day. The inevitable changes to routine (even when you minimize them) will be tiring all by themselves beyond what you factor in for walking and other physical activities.
- Longer trips are better than shorter ones. If we're going anywhere, we go for at least a week. This allows time to get used to new surroundings and changes in our routine. Weekend jaunts, with no time to get acclimated to someplace new, are not the ideal choice.
- Get your timing right. Schedule trips so that you won't be anywhere during "high season" or the holidays or any other time when crowds are at their peak. Early mornings are a particularly good time to travel, since there are fewer people up and about.
- Figure out how to keep at least some of your regular routine. The more you can maintain a business-as-usual schedule, the more comfortable a person with Alzheimer's will be. For example, follow your usual meal times and bedtime, and the usual bedtime rituals. Maybe catch a TV show you usually watch every week. Every little bit helps when your entire schedule has suddenly changed—you're not in your own

kitchen to eat, the coffee maker doesn't work the same, and the TV has a totally different remote.
- Whenever possible, make your new surroundings homelike by bringing a familiar pillow or blanket or a family picture to display in a hotel room. What helps the most will depend on what is important to the person with Alzheimer's.

Trip Insurance

We never bought trip insurance before Michael's diagnosis, and we haven't had to use what we've bought since then. But I appreciate the peace of mind that comes with knowing we can bow out if we need to, without losing much money. You don't always know what's going to happen with symptoms from day to day, much less looking weeks or months into the future, so you plan the best you can and, ideally, give yourself a little wiggle room with this sort of Plan B. I wouldn't plan a trip now without getting trip insurance.

Packing for Two

At this point I am in charge of packing for both Michael and me, but he and I always pack (and unpack) his things together. Even though he won't remember all the steps, I've learned that being part of the process still helps him be less anxious about his stuff.

Here are some things to keep in mind when you are packing:

- Pack as light as possible.

- Be sure to pack all prescription medications—but *not* in checked luggage. If you're flying, keep it in your carry-on. Lost baggage is always a risk, and getting new medication when you are out of town is *not* something you want to deal with.
- Make sure you bring your phone and charger. Actually, better make that make sure you bring chargers for *all* your various devices.
- Pack some familiar items to help improve orientation in a new place, and provide a feeling of security. A favorite blanket, maybe, or a couple family photos. We always bring a small whiteboard and erasable marker!
- Bring items for entertainment—books on tape, DVDs, magazines, music, whatever provides fun, calm or distraction, boredom-busting, and/or stress reduction. Think about what you might use en route as well as during your stay.
- Make copies of boarding passes, IDs, reservation confirmations, and the like to keep in your suitcase. If you misplace one en route…no problem! (If you are flying domestically, bring your passports anyway, as a backup to driver's license/state ID. The TSA is not going to be impressed with a photocopy!)
- Be sure to pack your patience!

When You're Flying

Michael and I have been frequent fliers for years, both for business (before we retired) and pleasure. Because it is such a familiar way to travel, it's still one of the easiest ways for us to go. Since Michael's diagnosis, we've relied on a few strategies to keep it as manageable as possible:

- Book seats on the bulkhead. More room is always good—it relieves the crowded feeling—and because it is close to the front of the plane you can exit ahead of most others and avoid the crush of people. I've learned that even if you can't choose bulkhead seats when reserving online, if you call the airline and explain you are traveling with someone with Alzheimer's, they will unblock the seats for you because they are considered disability seating. We have a doctor's note explaining that the front of the plane is best, and I carry a copy with me just in case I end up talking to someone at check-in who isn't that understanding.
- Check in and print boarding passes in advance, *before* you leave for the airport.
- Is someone picking you up at the airport? However you are traveling once you are off the plane, make arrangements (and confirm them) in advance so you don't end up in line for a cab, or trying to rent a car at peak periods. Apps like Uber can help, or a car service—prepaid means no muss, no fuss. Easier is always better.
- If you fly frequently, you can register with the TSA and avoid the long lines at security. This is a thing anyone can apply for (in other words, not a medical or Alzheimer's thing), but it is especially beneficial for a person dealing with Alzheimer's.
- When you go through security, hold your documents and IDs *and* those belonging to the person you are traveling with—otherwise, they are going to get misplaced. You may need to

explain to the TSA agent why you are doing this—they like everyone to hold their own.
- Tell the TSA agent when you are traveling with someone with Alzheimer's, and say you need to stay close and cannot be separated. They'll make special arrangements, usually without any fuss, so you can stick together.
- Put all important personal belongings in one bag—phone, wallet, ID, medication, and so on—to make it less likely you leave anything behind at security or on the plane. There's another good reason to have everything easily accessible: a person with Alzheimer's is likely to worry suddenly that important items like these have been stolen. You want to be able to reassure him or her by producing the items in question, without making any big deal about it.
- As you go through security, watch what your loved one takes out of bags or pockets and puts on the scanner, so you'll be able to help make sure everything is collected back up on the other side.
- If a bathroom break is needed, wait outside the door—airport layouts can be confusing, and it is too easy to get turned around and go the wrong way. If you need to go, wait until you are on the plane, if possible.
- At the gate, let the airline know you are traveling with a person with Alzheimer's and ask for early boarding. You can be among the first on the plane, which gives you extra time to get settled and organized, and avoids the crowd. Michael now gets a little agitated when we are getting on a plane, so the first that thing I do when we get to our seats is to get

out the iPod and headphones. Music is both calming and a distraction from whatever is disturbing the peace.
- You take the aisle seat. This way, you will be aware of coming and going should you nod off. And it'll be easier to communicate with the flight attendant, who should be informed of your loved one's condition. If anything comes up while in flight, it'll be easier if the flight attendant already knows your situation.
- Watch where your travel companion puts his or her belongings on the plane—overhead bin, under the seat, in their pockets, whatever—so you can check at the end of the flight to be sure everything comes off the plane with you.
- We have an adapter for our iPad that allows two people to plug in headphones at the same time so we can watch movies together—that's our favorite airplane pastime. Trust me on this: bring extra earbuds. They are easy to lose!

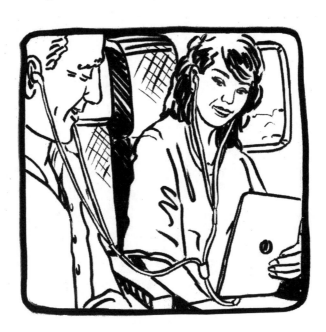

Car Travel

We have limited our drives to no longer than three hours because that seems to work best for us. Everyone is different, so it may take a little experience to figure out what's right for you.

The monotony of long drives tends to make Michael disengage, so my main strategy is to keep connected with him while we drive, by listening to music or playing car games, for example. (When I was a kid, my game was "Find that Car," and all I ever wanted to look for was the Volkswagen Beetle. But Michael and I, we go for trucks.) Sometimes we call people on the phone so we can talk to them together. Another idea is for your passenger to play the role of navigator (though you may have to define that loosely, depending on current abilities).

Or try that classic road-trip activity: talking. A person with Alzheimer's might not initiate a conversation, though, even if he or she enjoys participating in one, so it's up to you to figure out how to keep that particular ball in the air. In this situation, open-ended questions are *not* your friend. One good tactic is to reminisce—it allows you both to think happy thoughts, and reinforces memories. (More about this in Chapter 13: Be Interactive.)

Make car trips as efficient as possible, driving when you will miss rush hour, for example, and planning a route in advance. Include in your planning where you will make stops. If your trip is long enough to stop for a meal, choose a familiar place (i.e. a chain you know from home), and try to get there when it will be least crowded.

On the Road with Oliver

Having an emotional support animal along on a trip can be a great help. Having that responsibility, and the associated tasks, gives a person with Alzheimer's a positive focus and a feeling of being in control during a time when many things are shifting out of the usual routine. And, of course, an emotional support animal provides emotional support, and a feeling of security.

Traveling with a therapy dog also signals to the people nearby that the dog's person has some specific needs. When we travel with Oliver, I know I'm not going to have to start from square one with everyone I encounter to explain Michael's condition and how it might impact travel. People don't always need to know Michael's whole story, but just that he may need some accommodation, and that we are doing what we can to take care of it. Just having Oliver with us sends that message. Plus, flight attendants love Oliver!

On the other hand, traveling with Oliver adds another layer of work for me, so we don't always do it. (Of course leaving Oliver at home adds another task to my to-do list: who will take care of Oliver? So, like everything else, it's a balance.)

Part of whether we travel with our dog depends on how we are traveling. It's simple enough to put Oliver in the car with us, but there's still the question of whether our target destination, and intermediate stops, will be dog-friendly. Flying with an animal is a more challenging undertaking, but because flying is a stressful way to travel, Michael needs Oliver more. The main thing to keep in mind if you want to fly with an emotional support animal is to plan well in advance. Register your animal with the airlines as soon as you get your tickets. Most airlines require a signed letter from your loved one's doctor before a support animal will be allowed to travel on the plane, and the airline can provide a sample of what this letter should contain. Bring a copy of that signed letter when you go, in case you get asked for proof at the airport.

Roll with It

Traveling with a person with Alzheimer's requires patience and flexibility: learn to roll with it. Even when things get hairy, you have to stay calm, cool, and collected because that prevents things from getting even hairier. This is true whether you are confronted with an inflexible TSA agent or a rude fellow traveler—or your loved one's anxiety. Do whatever you need to do to keep yourself calm until the difficult moment passes. If you stay positive, so will your loved one. And probably the snippy person behind the desk too.

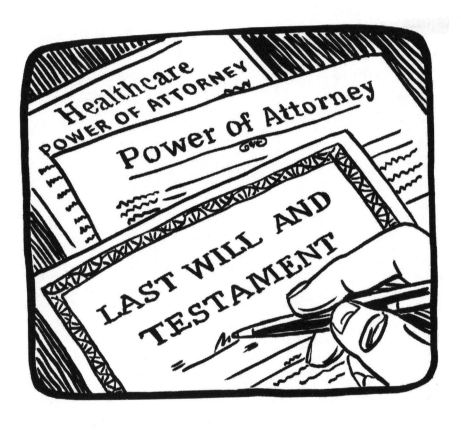

CHAPTER 16

BE PROACTIVE: LEGAL, FINANCIAL, AND LONG-TERM CARE PLANNING

Looking into the future can be frightening after an Alzheimer's diagnosis. Understandably, it can be tempting to put it out of your mind, making it easier to avoid unpleasant tasks like making a will, researching long-term care options, and creating power-of-attorney documents.

But you know what's even scarier than facing what the future might bring? Arriving in that future *with no plan for managing it.*

You're dealing with a disease with no cure, so the future is daunting, period. Thinking about the future can't change what's going to happen. But neither can *not* thinking about it. The only way to get any control over what happens in the future is to figure out what you want your life to look like given the situation you are in, what supports you need to make that life happen, and how to get those supports. You need a plan. Your family *needs* you to have a plan. Having a plan empowers people to help you effectively.

You also need positivity. I'm not saying it's easy to maintain hope when you stare down the realities of Alzheimer's, but you *have* to find a way.

One of the best ways to stay positive is to make a plan and prepare as best you can for whatever comes. The more proactive and prepared you are, the better off you'll be, and the more in control of the situation you will feel.

It's Never Too Soon to Get Your Affairs in Order
I asked Matt Field, head of Right at Home, the caregiver agency we use, about the most common mistakes families have made by the time they end up in his office. I thought he'd say something like, "trying to do too much on their own." But without a moment's hesitation, he said the most common issue was not having their affairs in order. They come to him for help with a cognitively impaired loved one and don't yet know who has power of attorney, who makes the medical decisions, who controls the finances. If he could give everybody one piece of advice before *he met them professionally, he said, it would be to take care of all medical and legal planning issues immediately upon diagnosis. Anything not yet done needs to be done, and anything done previously needs to be reviewed with the Alzheimer's diagnosis in mind.*

You Need Professional Help
Don't feel you should take on legal and financial planning tasks by yourself. Taking care of a person with Alzheimer's is mentally exhausting, so you need to recognize the things that are above your "pay grade" and let someone else handle them. Therefore don't be afraid to ask for that help. And if you can afford it, don't be afraid to pay for someone else's expertise. These are things worth having done, and done right, and worth paying for. Basic guidance from

legal and financial professionals will pay for itself in many cases. Low- or no-cost options are most likely available in your community too. Check with your local senior center, often a great source of resources and support.

Assemble a Team

You are going to be like a general contractor, pulling together a number of specialists to work on particular tasks and coordinating their work as necessary to keep things moving smoothly and get things completed.

You may already have done this with a healthcare team, leaning on some combination of internist, neurologist, geriatrician, and specialists for any other conditions you are managing. Maybe there's a nurse practitioner or PA in there somewhere, and/or a psychologist or social worker. If this is the case, then you already know how important it is to establish and maintain communication with—and among—your medical team.

Now it's time to create a team of legal and financial professionals who also will communicate with each other. You'll want to do whatever you can to facilitate connections between the lawyers, financial planners, insurance agents, accountants, and bankers on your team. Sharing paperwork also is vital, especially the power-of-attorney documents.

These new players may not all need to interface with the healthcare team, but some information will need to move back and forth, and you will play the lead and messenger in some cases. You definitely will want to ask your doctor to provide a letter certifying that the person with Alzheimer's is fully capable of revising a will or making decisions regarding the contents of an advance directive. Once you receive the letter, you'll give it to the financial and/or legal professional assisting you. Keep a copy for yourself so that anyone can see the validity of the letter at the time it was created and signed. This makes it easier to validate the illness and demonstrate that those with the disease have the capacity to make these important decisions for themselves.

Add a trusted advisor—a friend—to your team. Mine is Anne Garr. Anne is both a close friend and our personal attorney, with Freeborn & Peters LLP of Chicago. You need someone who is a sounding board when things get emotional.

Remember: *you* are the captain of this team. In addition to the intangible and emotional components associated with Alzheimer's, a variety of fees are involved when using consultants. Therefore, it's in your best interest to take this managerial role seriously. Choose a team you can rely on, but never let go of control entirely.

Work Together as Much as Possible, as Soon as Possible

It is critical to obtain input from the person with the disease. This is true for just about everything, though especially important when it comes to legal and financial issues. My recommendation? Plan together and do it now.

Because of the changing nature of Alzheimer's, it's important to plan for the future as soon as possible. If you can begin this process following the diagnosis, even better. Knowing there is a plan in place is just as good for relieving some anxiety about the future for the person with the diagnosis as it is for the caregivers(s). Caregivers benefit from knowing a plan is in place. A plan that reflects the wishes of the person with Alzheimer's also gives caretakers some peace of mind. Whenever decision-making is shared, the level of stress can be reduced.

Michael and I completed a significant portion of our financial planning before we got married and during his heart-related health scare. Still, when Alzheimer's came into our life, it brought with it new issues we needed to address, or address sooner than we'd thought we'd need to. And it meant we wanted to revise some of the plans we had already put into place (which we did by going back to the same wonderful estate attorney, Elizabeth Garlovsky).

Prior to Michael's diagnosis or "BA" (before Alzheimer's), Michael used to manage our finances. It's not that I couldn't or wouldn't take care of finances, but from the list of tasks that kept our life together moving along, this one fell to him. So I had to get up to speed on all things financial and put myself in the driver's seat. We worked together as much as we could, talking over all the important points, sharing ideas, opinions, and strategies, but Michael's challenges meant he could no longer manage these responsibilities. Still, Michael has been a part of all meetings, and it's only recently that the challenges of the illness have impacted his big-picture understanding of our business and personal finances.

That wasn't an easy transition for either of us, since a big part of Michael's identity has always been his business acumen. I'm mentioning this because I want you to know it can be done. If you are not 100 percent confident in the role, consider hiring a professional. You should never be afraid to ask for help. And whatever you do, don't let uncertainty about how to handle things prevent you from taking action as soon as possible.

Financial Planning

Hopefully, you have already put some financial plans in place for retirement. If you haven't, please start now and with Alzheimer's in mind. Here's why: the person with Alzheimer's may be retiring earlier than planned; plus a caregiver might need significant time off—I used Family Medical Leave Act (FMLA) time off to care for Michael early on. Or, like me, caregivers may end up retiring early themselves. If you are retired, you will undoubtedly add some Alzheimer's-related expenses to your life. Whichever path you take, there will be significant financial consequences. Ignoring them in hopes they go away may seem appealing, but I promise you that's not going to work. Go ahead and deal with the financial situation; it's always better to be informed.

Financial planning is about your needs and your goals and how you will pay for them. A reputable financial planner can help you figure out how best to afford the care necessary for a person with Alzheimer's, when and how to file for Social Security and other relevant government benefits, and what types and amounts of insurance you need (and don't need). They can help you determine how far employee benefits, retirement accounts, and savings will take you, and how well insured you are (or aren't). If you need or want investment advice, seek out a financial planner who specializes in that niche, but only select someone with whom you can clearly communicate. It's critical that you can understand and follow the process.

A financial planner can help you navigate the following areas:

- Medicare
- Medicare drug benefit (plan D)
- Veteran's benefits

- Medicaid
- Social Security
- Social Security disability (for people under 65)
- Social Security SSI (supplemental security income)
- Long-term care insurance
- Updating the beneficiaries on all your accounts to be appropriate choices now

Financial Vulnerability

When Matt Field of Right at Home points out the importance of having a financial power of attorney (POA) in place as early as possible, he emphasizes that cognitive decline makes people extremely vulnerable to financial exploitation. Too many families have already learned this the hard way by the time they meet Matt, so it's a message he hopes will get to people sooner in the process. It is common for those with Alzheimer's to be targeted by unscrupulous telemarketers or shady home repair people or phony charities, but the danger is most often closer to home. Sadly, some caregivers and family members can become extremely exploitive.

Attorney Kerry Peck agrees; he says that it's often someone who knows the person with Alzheimer's. This victimization occurs in different guises, but lawyers can help. Attorneys who specialize in this area can help freeze assets in the midst of a problem, though it's always better to take preventative action. Financial exploitation may be straight-out theft or another complicated form of swindling, but the solution is the same: have someone you trust closely monitoring the financial life of your loved one with Alzheimer's; put a financial POA in place; work with financial professionals to establish safeguards (i.e., work with a financial institution to make sure a caregiver is unable to bring another individual into a bank in order to withdraw funds from your accounts).

Every family has to deal with this kind of financial safety in ways that make sense for them. For Michael and me, switching financial affairs to my plate pretty early on was a difficult but beneficial process, and we've been able to avoid problems like these by using our legal and financial advisors to make a strong, enforceable plan. It's not a transition anyone wants to make, but I think everyone with Alzheimer's would be well served to choose a person who can be trusted to take over finances, right down to reviewing checking and credit card accounts weekly so any problems that appear can be addressed immediately, before they become a serious issue or beyond repair. Remember, it's about putting your team in place and allowing your team and trusted advisor to help you through these difficult times in your new normal.

Talk to a Lawyer

I might *still* be on the phone with the government, buried in a pile of paperwork, if I hadn't gotten an attorney to sort out Social Security disability. It is the best $600 I have ever spent. The lawyer filled out all the application forms with me and reviewed Michael's medical records. He walked me through the process, which I found baffling and overwhelming without his help. I don't know how anyone ever files for disability *without* expert advice.

A lawyer is an important part of your professional planning team. Look for a "generation" attorney or an elder law and estate planning firm. If you are lucky, you will find an attorney or firm that specializes in Alzheimer's planning, though that's not strictly necessary.

Nonetheless, you'll want a lawyer to help you with:

- Power of attorney (which might also be called a "power of attorney for property"). This type of POA designates a person to manage finances and make financial decisions for people with Alzheimer's at the point where they can no longer reliably handle those things themselves.
- Healthcare power of attorney (yes, it's a different document). A healthcare POA designates a person to make medical decisions for those with Alzheimer's who can't effectively manage them on their own.
- Will. If the person with Alzheimer's doesn't have one, get one ASAP. If there is already a will in place, have it reviewed for any necessary or desired changes after an Alzheimer's diagnosis.
- Revocable Trusts. Occasionally, these documents make sense in addition to a financial power of attorney, depending on the kind of assets involved.

You may also want legal help with:

- Medicare planning
- Social Security and disability

- Insurance
- Healthcare options
- Preserving financial assets while paying for long-term care
- Long-term plans for living arrangements

I became Michael's POA for financial, legal, and health issues prior to our wedding, since we were already dealing with some health issues before the Alzheimer's diagnosis. That came after we were married.

One of the most important things you can do for people with Alzheimer's is to help them get their health and financial plans *in writing* as soon as possible. The course of the disease is unpredictable, and you want to officially capture their wishes while they are still technically competent to sign off on them. This should bring everyone some peace of mind, especially those with the disease but you as well. It will ease the burden of taking over medical and legal responsibility in the future. The right documents, properly executed, will enable you to proceed with the confidence that you are conducting business in the way your loved one would want, even after it cannot be expressed to you directly.

Regardless of how you approach legal and financial matters, you'll want to establish clear communication about the process with close family and maybe even some good friends. This, too, should happen in the process as early as possible and whenever subsequent changes are made. That way, no one is surprised. Everyone who potentially will be affected by the decisions needs to be in the loop from the start—while the person with Alzheimer's is still capable of discussing his or her wishes. If these issues don't arise until a crisis hits, the situation is open to second-guessing, misunderstanding, and hurt feelings. For example, the doctor's office is not the place to hold your first discussion about who has (or doesn't have) medical power of attorney. You want to have these things out in the open *before* it's strictly necessary. That gives your family the best chance to discuss issues rationally and calmly. No one makes the best decision or argument when emotions are running wild. And when it comes to abiding by a person's plans, nobody gains by secrecy or fighting. People's feelings may get hurt and you could be the topic of gossip, but that's their issue, not yours. Your energy should be focused on your loved one.

Elizabeth Garlovsky, Estate Planning Attorney

Some people are hesitant about choosing someone to be their POA because they fear making a choice (one child over another, for example) will cause family conflict. In my professional experience, though, I can tell you that lack of documentation, or documentation that's ambiguous, is far more likely to lead to family discord. This is especially true in blended families, but in any family each person may well have different ideas and goals as to what is "supposed" to happen. The only person whose opinion really counts in this is the person who is making the POA and related documents and plans.

Your best bet, therefore, is to put your wishes in writing, getting it done carefully and correctly, and then be smart about communicating to all the relevant people what your choices are and why. Talking with your loved ones, being as transparent as possible, is the only reliable way to avoid a mess. This includes talking to people who don't have an official role (for example, who are not your POA but might feel they could be).

Laws vary from state to state—one of the reasons you should have professional guidance—but the key component of getting plans done carefully and correctly is documenting a person's capacity (in the legal sense) to sign off on a document. This safeguards the plan against questions from disgruntled family members or other loved ones. When I do these documents for a client, I often rely on a client's neurological evaluation and the evaluating doctor's determination of his or her "testamentary capacity." A letter in your file from the treating medical professional, concurrent with any legal or financial work you are doing, is invaluable. In some situations, it might make sense to have a video of a person signing the documents, with witnesses—whether or not the witnesses are required by state law.

An attorney with specialization in estate planning can help with this and the many other strands that have to come together properly to make sure things unfold over time the way a person with Alzheimer's wants them to; this is true whether the goals were established before or after the diagnosis. Too many people allow their discomfort about talking about these things stop them from taking action. The urge to put it off is almost universal. But what is also universal is the huge feeling of relief once it is done. It's an anxiety-filled process, but judging by my clients, everyone feels less anxious once it is done.

Kerry Peck, attorney and co-author of
Alzheimer's and the Law: Counseling Clients
with Dementia and Their Families

Who do you want to make the most important decisions in your life when you can't? A trusted loved one? The courts? If you don't designate someone to be your POA, you could be headed for a protracted court battle over "guardianship" of you and your resources. What's even worse is that your family will be dragged through a difficult process when they are already in a high-stress or even crisis situation.

In other words: draw up your documents and do it now. Fighting this out, among family and/or in the courts, is emotional, expensive, and avoidable. Unfortunately, the nature of this disease is that at some point a person is going to become unable to independently make the decisions legally—and no one wants that. The best defense is to decide for yourself who will decide for you when it comes to that. The best decisions about your future will be the ones made by you. Be proactive.

Care Planning

The third area in which advance planning is crucial might be the one that's hardest, emotionally, to consider. What kind of care will a person with Alzheimer's need or want, and how will that care be arranged for and managed? As with financial and legal matters, don't allow yourself to get in your own way. Just do it. Look into the future, knowing there really isn't any crystal ball to show you clearly what will happen, and make the best plan you can. Strive for that balance between a positive attitude and being prepared for whatever may come.

I know it's not easy. Even as I drove to a memory care center for an informational tour, I thought I might not be able to walk inside. On the other hand, I would rather know what's ahead than keep myself in the dark. Knowledge really is power; that's my motto. I've always planned on being Michael's primary caregiver myself. I've handled it this far, and I don't plan to change it. But I needed to understand our options. What if we did need a different kind of care? In the meantime, maybe I could learn something that would further help me help Michael. The professionals in this field have told me that sometimes living outside the home becomes a better option for a person with Alzheimer's. They added that this particular memory care center (Silverado—see below) is the best. A friend whose mother is there helped me realize I should look into how the place works. So I decided to go. I knew I didn't need to make any decisions on that visit or change any plans. But I did need to keep an open mind and see what I could learn.

Building Brain Connections
The person who showed me around Silverado in Highland Park, Illinois, is Liz Lindeman, MSW, Director of Resident and Family Services. Part of what makes Silverado a positive place to be for people with Alzheimer's, she explained to me, is their "Nexus" program for those with the earlier stages of dementias. Nexus means "connections" in Latin. Silverado works toward making connections in the brain to slow progression of Alzheimer's and similar diseases. To build and maintain brain activity, the Nexus program combines several components, including exercise, stress reduction, social activities, and cognitive exercise to stimulate the intellect.

So Silverado uses music and art therapy, storytelling exercises, support groups, writing, trivia games, clubs—anything and everything that jogs the mind; provides purposeful, meaningful activity;

focuses on current abilities; uses language; and engages people with others and with the world.

I wish the same could be said of all facilities, but there's still a ways to go until we're in that world, and this is one of the reasons doing your homework in advance is so important. But personally, I was also happy to see professionals and experts putting their faith behind the same sort of approach that's meant so much to me and Michael.

As with other types of planning discussed in this chapter, talking to loved ones is a crucial part of the process. To get the kind of long-term care that is best for people with Alzheimer's is to ask for their opinion. Find out their wishes, preferences, concerns, and goals. Michael and I have discussed the situation many, many times.

Talk about end-of-life care issues as well as living arrangements and types of care. Do it even though these are hard conversations. Then do it some more: all loved ones with a stake in this can and should be included in conversations about the future. It will be worth it in the long run. Later, when decision-making becomes more difficult, you will, hopefully, have some peace of mind in knowing your loved one's preferences.

These kinds of talks should include all the paperwork discussed in this chapter. It is also important to discuss, and discuss again, the things that aren't likely to end up in a legal document. But the details of care, over the long term, are as important as bank accounts and other areas. Liz Lindeman at Silverado points out that most families wait for some kind of "sign" to show them it is time to make the jump to moving their loved one with Alzheimer's into a facility.

For some people this time might never come, but for many it takes the drastic shape of slipping in the shower and spending a long time alone before help arrives, or a hospital stay following a preventable injury from a fall down the stairs.

Research and plan for care early on, *before* you need it. This is the best way to avoid a traumatic incident that puts everyone into crisis mode. An emergency move-in is never the best way to make a transition. Instead of waiting until something really big and bad happens, take note of small changes. For example, has a formerly laid-back person recently become aggressive? Is he or she refusing to cooperate with a caregiver on basic self-care, like washing up, for an extended period of time? Has it become apparent that your loved one can no longer manage personal hygiene?

That day at the memory care center, I did manage to walk right in. It was a painful meeting, though. I felt like the wind had been knocked out of me. And I was right that Michael didn't need to come with me. But it was an important meeting nonetheless. I am planning for the two of us to continue living together, no matter how difficult it gets. I'm confident we'll find a way. But I also will continue to explore all options so that when decision points come—and with this disease, you just never know exactly when that will happen—I'll be prepared to make informed choices alongside my team.

CHAPTER 17

LIVING THE 24-HOUR RULE: YOUR NEW NORMAL

We want this book to provide a wide range of strategies that will help people create their own "new normal" with a high quality of life and the ability to preserve your life for as long as possible. Remember, there is no one right way to do this, and there is no one strategy that will work for everyone or work all the time or, unfortunately, work forever. Still, it's important that you try any and every potential strategy to see what works best for you.

Regardless of where you are on this challenging journey, the book is designed to meet you there. So start with the chapter that's right for you. Maybe you'll begin at the beginning or at the end or somewhere in between. It doesn't matter. What does matter is reading about the strategies that will help you *now*. Stay with the tips and strategies that work, and disregard what doesn't work; you might come back to something later when you need it most. This is your book, your journey, your life. Keep trying new and different things so you'll build an ever-better array of strategies to have on tap. Keep in mind that this won't happen all at once; it doesn't need to. The goal is to provide options that empower versus overwhelm.

Here is your checklist of specific action items to help you put into motion as easily as possible the creative and helpful strategies presented in the previous chapters. They can be summarized into a few broad themes, which should all sound familiar by this point:

Routine is key. Having a schedule for each day and each week makes everything easier for people with Alzheimer's—and for their caregivers.

But remain flexible. Ironically, routines are intended to infuse consistency, but we all know that life isn't so neat sometimes, so you have to be nimble and willing to go with the flow. Furthermore, what works today might not work tomorrow, but it might work again another day. Not every strategy or activity is going to appeal to everyone, or even apply. Choose and adapt strategies according to your circumstances and the specific personalities involved. Think of the 24-Hour Rule program as one that differs from person to person and constantly evolves.

Three P's: Be Proactive, Be Prepared, Be Positive. Taking action is the essence of the 24-Hour Rule. Yes, you should feel your feelings and acknowledge your emotions. You've got 24 hours. Then take action. Be proactive. Plan for the future, even if it's not the future you wanted: be prepared for whatever comes your way. If you can, find a way to stay positive even in the face of an uncertain future and a present no one chooses. Combine all the love, empathy, understanding, patience, and sense of humor you can muster. That will be your way of getting through. Sometimes it will be all about your attitude.

Be an advocate. Advocate for your loved one, first and foremost. But also advocate for 1) ridding Alzheimer's of its stigma, 2) educating the public and decision-makers about the disease and its consequences, and 3) finding and promoting short- and long-term solutions.

Embrace variety. The best way to stimulate all parts of the brain is to engage in all sorts of activities. Select multiple pursuits each day, choose from a range of activities, and try mixing and matching different types of stimuli depending upon where you are and what's available. Maybe something is mentally challenging and social like an art class. Or you may discover fun and fine-motor-skills-boosting activities like Jenga. One day you might choose something more physical, like riding a bike or power-walking outdoors. Choose anything and everything that keeps your loved one active and engaged.

Checklist

Plan for the Future

- [ ] Assemble a team of professionals; make any appointments with your financial and legal advisors that are necessary.
- [ ] Complete power-of-attorney documents for financial and medical decision-making.
- [ ] Communicate your plans to your family.
- [ ] Keep lines of communication open in order to keep family and friends informed and relevant medical professionals in the loop.
- [ ] Shift responsibilities for finances as necessary.

- ☐ Document the preferences of the person with Alzheimer's for financial, legal, and medical matters.
- ☐ Research memory care facilities and other options, so that you don't have to make high-stakes decisions under pressure or in an extreme emotional state.

Get Organized

- ☐ Acquire extras of all-important items—extra set of keys, extra wallet, and so on. Keep them handy.
- ☐ Establish a routine—daily and weekly.
- ☐ Get a whiteboard (or two) and find an ideal place to set it up.
- ☐ Establish a schedule for the day and post it on the whiteboard. Aim for a day that's full but not *busy*.
- ☐ Get and hang a BIG calendar.
- ☐ Make a set of laminated cards to make key information easy to carry and find.
- ☐ Set up a good filing system; use an "active" folder for current information you might need on tap.
- ☐ Create or update a list of passwords for all important accounts. Stash one for quick reference and store a couple copies very carefully, including at least one with a trusted person who can keep it somewhere outside your home.
- ☐ Make copies of all key documents and distribute to key people.
- ☐ Switch to digital clocks and watches.
- ☐ Make a list of contact names and numbers.
- ☐ Create a charging "station" at home, and establish a routine about when to plug in so you never have to worry about dead phones.

- [ ] Organize your closet back to basics, so that getting dressed is easy and less frustrating.
- [ ] Know all the places where your loved one tends to set stuff down and put things away.

"Proof" the Home

- [ ] Get a professional assessment of home safety or conduct a thorough one yourself, looking for worst-case scenarios. Include cleaning and personal care items, foods, and clothing as well as the rooms, doors, windows, and furniture.
- [ ] Address risks identified in home safety survey.
- [ ] De-clutter.
- [ ] Update home maintenance.
- [ ] Order/wear ID jewelry systems like Life Alert.
- [ ] Set your home alarms system, if you have one, to optimal settings.
- [ ] Set up a safe system for storing, remembering, and safely dispensing medication.
- [ ] Make or update a list of all medications with names, doses, prescribing doctor, and condition treated.
- [ ] Get to know your pharmacist.

See Your Doctor

- [ ] See your doctor(s). Make regular medical appointments. Take care of any and all general health issues, and, of course, follow advice on Alzheimer's, including the use of medications.

- ☐ Discuss any changes you make to your lifestyle, including diet and exercise.

Exercise

- ☐ Schedule exercise into your day and week.
- ☐ Enjoy a favorite form of exercise, something you do regularly or used to love to do.
- ☐ Try a new kind of exercise; find out what else you enjoy.
- ☐ Mix it up; in your exercise schedule, find time for different types of activities.
- ☐ Sign up for a class or individual instruction, or call on a friend with experience to teach you a new kind of fitness.
- ☐ Talk to instructors, trainers, gym staff, workout buddies, and anyone else you can think of about Alzheimer's and the effects it has on your loved one and how they can help.

Eat Right

- ☐ Post a list of brain-healthy foods in your kitchen to help in planning meals and making shopping lists.
- ☐ Clear from your kitchen any foods you don't want to include in your brain-healthy lifestyle.
- ☐ Make a shopping list and stock up on essential items for the MIND, like almonds, green tea, and olive oil.
- ☐ Schedule time to shop for perishables (fish, produce, etc.) at least once a week.

Find a "Buddy"

- ☐ Look into home healthcare agencies.
- ☐ Reach out to local organizations that might provide volunteer help, like your religious organization, if you belong to one, or a senior center or university.
- ☐ Ask if anyone is using the "buddy" model; if not, explain it to agencies and organizations, and they may be able to provide someone who fits the mold—even if it's a new idea.
- ☐ Talk honestly with friends and family members to see what help they can/will provide; the "buddy" role may be an appealing way to help out, but you may need to explain how it works. If someone voices interest, ask for a commitment with respect to time and schedule.

Consider an Emotional Support Animal

- ☐ If you want to make room in your life for an emotional support animal, do some research to determine which animal is best for your situation.
- ☐ Get appropriate training for you and your animal.
- ☐ If an animal does not fit realistically into your life, consider other ways to experience that kind of nurturing, companionship, and unconditional love, like befriending someone else's pet; even watching a fish tank or birds at a feeder is calming.

Socialize

- ☐ Reach out to someone you'd like to connect or reconnect with and make a plan to see him or her.
- ☐ Schedule social activities regularly.

Look Good

- ☐ Set up a whiteboard to use for personal care reminders.
- ☐ Establish a regular routine for managing personal care.
- ☐ Review safety of personal care products and processes. Switch regular razors for electric, for example, and remove rarely used products before they can cause trouble.

Deal with Driving

- ☐ Discuss driving and plans for stopping driving.
- ☐ Get a driving safety evaluation.
- ☐ Investigate alternate forms of transportation and make plans for how your loved one will travel once driving is no longer an option. Find out what's available in terms of public transportation, car service, taxis, apps like Uber, senior transportation services, and volunteer drivers from local organizations. Assess accessibility, safety, and cost. Remember to compare against cost of buying, maintaining, and insuring a car; taxis may not seem so expensive once you do the research. Don't forget to consider walking and biking as possible forms of transportation.

Get Creative

- ☐ Make a list of creative activities you would like to try. Include old favorites ("I used to love to draw"), bucket list items ("I've always wanted to play drums"), and activities you might like to do with someone else ("I wonder if my friend would go to a knitting class with me").
- ☐ Sign up for a class, private lessons, or a club to explore one or more of the above.
- ☐ Choose a DIY art project of whatever kind. You can wing it or seek guidance from the library or YouTube. Remember, it can be something humble like paint-by-numbers or a simple craft project. Check out Toys "R" Us.
- ☐ Put creative activities on your regular schedule.
- ☐ Attend performances, listen to music at home, visit a gallery or museum, or just page through an art book or a beautifully designed magazine.

Be an Advocate

- ☐ Tell or update others about Alzheimer's, its effects on you and your loved one, and explain how they can help you personally as well as generate awareness about the disease.
- ☐ Sign up to participate in an event designed to raise awareness and/or funds.
- ☐ Sign up online to receive notices of opportunities for activism with your local Alzheimer's Association.
- ☐ Research possible clinical trials.

Communicate

- Help friends communicate in effective ways. For example, instead of posing open-ended questions like, "What did you do today?" ask, "Did you play golf or tennis today?"
- Try gentle coaching with people who are afraid or unsure about how best to interact with a person suffering from Alzheimer's; share your strategies.

Work Your Brain

- Create a memory montage; maybe it can even be a joint project. Work on it when you can. Review photos and other memorabilia together or listen to old favorite songs that remind you of special times in your lives.
- Schedule specific "fun" times into your day and week.
- Pull some games out of the back of the closet, or pick up a few new ones. Keep them easily accessible, somewhere in sight so that you'll actually play them. Try enough different games to figure out your favorites. Which ones work best as distractions? Which ones are best for groups? Which ones encourage socializing or practice other skills?
- Plan a way to get laughs into your daily life. Your own sense of humor and attitude are great places to start. Still, make an effort to schedule time for a "movie date" to watch a classic comedy or invite a friend to come play your own zany brand of ping-pong or cards.

- ☐ Schedule outings of any and all kinds—a walk around the block or to the next porch over to visit with a neighbor, even a simple errand will do. Whatever engages you in the wider world in a non-stressful way is good.
- ☐ Assign chores. Choose something that matches ability and, if possible, interest.
- ☐ Subscribe to some magazines and/or newspapers and become a regular at your library so you always have something to read or watch that captures your interest.
- ☐ Try your hand at crossword puzzles or any other mentally challenging activity you can dream up—and enjoy. The more variety, the better.

Caregivers, Take Good Care of Yourself

- ☐ Schedule "you" time into each day for exercise, hobbies, or just grabbing a coffee with your friend.
- ☐ See your doctor regularly to manage your overall health.
- ☐ Enlist professionals, volunteers, friends, and family to help you provide care, including giving you time off to nurture yourself.
- ☐ Stay engaged in your own life, relationships, interests, and goals—schedule time to do so and get backup care to allow it.
- ☐ Consider working with a therapist and/or support group for caregivers.

It is a great gift to your loved one, as well as to yourself, if you can create a life lived fully now. That there is no cure for Alzheimer's does *not* mean your life should stop. No cure does *not* mean no hope, no joy, or no love. Walking the fine line of accepting what you can't change while making positive changes where possible is what the 24-Hour Rule is all about.

It's a long journey, and like every other path, it begins by taking one step. That first step doesn't get you all the way there, but you will never arrive if you don't begin. Why not pick one thing from this book to put into action today? Then do that again the next day, and the next. That's what I do every day. That's how you'll get to your new normal.

RESOURCES

Lee S. Freedman, MD, internal medicine—www.mdvip.com/leefreedmanmd

Julie Fohrman, MA, MAG GCM, Gerontologist, Founder and Principal of North Shore Geriatric Care— julie@northshoregeriatric.com; www.northshoregeriatric.com

Amanda G. Smith, MD, Medical Director, University of South Florida Health Byrd Alzheimer's Institute—asmith2@health.usf.edu; www.health.usf.edu/byrd/

Jill Smith, MA, CCRC, Assistant Director for Clinical Research, USF Health Byrd Alzheimer's Institute—jsmith10@health.usf.edu

Dr. Chad J. Yucus, MD, Neurologist, Glenview, IL, NorthShore Neurology, NorthShore University Health System—www.northshore.org/neurological-institute

Linda Randall, PHD—leviasue@aol.com

Kerry Peck, Esq., Managing Partner, Peck Ritchey LLC, Chicago Elder Law Litigation Lawyers, Guardianship—www.peckbloom.com

Elizabeth A. Garlovsky, Esq., Robbins, Salomon & Pratt, Ltd., Estate Planning—egarlovsky@rsplaw.com; www.rsplaw.com/

Erica Hornthal, MA, LCPC, BC-DMT, Chicago Dance Therapy—www.chicagodancetherapy.com

Noah Plotkin, Life Rhythms, Inc. Music Therapy—noah@liferhythemsinc.com; www.liferhythmsinc.com/

Martha Clare Morris, PHD, Rush University Medical Center, author of *The MIND Diet*—www.rush.edu/news/diet-may-help-prevent-alzheimers

Carol Ross, CDBA, Owner and Director of Training for the Northern Chicago Region Canine Dimensions—carolr@CanineDimensions.com; www.CanineDimensions.com

Matt Field, Principal, Right At Home Care—matt@rightathomesnsc.com; www.rightathome.net

Liz Lindeman, MSW, Director of Resident and Family Services, Silverado Alzheimer's Memory Care Center—elindeman@silveradocare.com; www.silveradocare.com

NOTES

NOTES

NOTES

NOTES

NOTES

NOTES

NOTES

NOTES

NOTES

NOTES

Made in the USA
Charleston, SC
30 October 2016